T0341792

The short guide to mental health

Deirdre Heenan and Jennifer Betts

First published in Great Britain in 2025 by

Policy Press, an imprint of
Bristol University Press
University of Bristol
1–9 Old Park Hill
Bristol
BS2 8BB
UK
t: +44 (0)117 374 6645
e: bup-info@bristol.ac.uk

Details of international sales and distribution partners are available at policy.bristoluniversitypress.co.uk

British Library Cataloguing in Publication Data
A catalogue record for this book is available from the British Library

ISBN 978-1-4473-5244-0 paperback
ISBN 978-1-4473-5249-5 ePub
ISBN 978-1-4473-7034-5 ePdf

Cover design: Qube Design
Front cover image: iStock
Bristol University Press and Policy Press use environmentally responsible print partners.
Printed and bound in Great Britain by CPI Group (UK) Ltd, Croydon, CR0 4YY

Contents

List of figures, tables and boxes

Figures

Tables

Boxes

Introduction: Why mental health matters

In our rapidly changing world, understanding mental health has never been more important. The term 'mental health' is not new, but it is frequently misunderstood and misrepresented. Historically, due to stigma and fear, there has been a reluctance to discuss mental health. It has fallen behind physical health in terms of attention, research and funding and has been conspicuously absent from wider debates about the National Health Service (NHS). While perceptions are changing, there is still much work to do. It is now generally accepted that there is much more to good health than a physically healthy body. Most would agree that a healthy mind is equally important. Mental health is often described as being on a continuum – on one end is the healthy point and at the other end is the ill point – with many varying experiences along this continuum.

Following years of underinvestment and lack of attention globally, mental health services are now firmly on the agenda in many countries, including the UK, and there has been a sea change in public attitudes. However, there is still a long way to go. A long-term commitment to investment and reform is needed to expand access to mental health services and support vital improvements in the quality of care experienced by people using these services (The King's Fund, 2019).

The need for action on mental health is indisputable and urgent. Good mental health is crucial to overall health and wellbeing. The COVID-19 pandemic and associated lockdowns in the UK between March 2020 and mid-2021 worsened an already alarming situation. Since the early 1990s, mental health services have undergone a radical transformation, with the development of community-based, multidisciplinary alternatives to hospitals and asylums. Although there have been significant advancements in our knowledge and understanding in this field, there are still major issues in terms of access to services and investment in this area of healthcare. In 2011, the government acknowledged the large treatment gap for people with mental health issues and promised to deliver 'parity of esteem' between mental and physical health services (Baker and Gheera, 2020). In practice though, the lack of funding that mental health services receive in comparison to other health services and the low priority afforded to it mean that it remains very much a 'Cinderella service'. Despite repeated commitments and pledges to transform and improve the quality and quantity of services, progress has been painfully slow. COVID-19 propelled mental health up the political agenda and government promised more funding. However, while these commitments are welcome, it will take more than money to address long-standing policy and practice issues.

The World Health Organization (WHO) frames mental health in terms of fundamental human rights:

> Mental health is a basic human right for all people. Everyone, whoever they are, has a right to the highest attainable standard of mental health. This includes the right to be protected from mental health risks, the right to available, accessible, and good quality care, and the right to liberty, independence and inclusion in the community. (WHO, 2022c, p 1)

Prior to the 1960s, a severe mental illness was generally accompanied with a dire prognosis. Expectations of leading a normal life were low, and individuals were discouraged from engaging in education, employment, personal relationships and independent living. This negative, paternalistic view was challenged by the concept of recovery (WHO, 2022c). While this term is associated with an array of models and definitions, it is usually associated with individual agency, autonomy and empowerment. People can, and do, recover from mental ill health. There is a significant body of evidence that demonstrates that improving outcomes for people with mental health problems supports enhanced wellbeing, builds resilience and independence, and optimises life chances, as well as reducing premature mortality (Drake et al, 2014; Whitley et al, 2015). Across the UK, there is increasing support for progressive community-based models of mental health that support human rights, are delivered locally and focus on prevention and early intervention. It is essential that the approach to mental health and equality is fit for the 21st century, with care being delivered close to home, technological advances being understood and embraced, and asset-based approaches being considered to minimise the 'deficits' that people can experience.

The WHO have published extensively on mental health, seeing 'the promotion, protection and restoration of mental health ... as a vital concern of individuals, communities and societies throughout the world' (WHO, nd). In their 'Mental health' fact sheet, the WHO describe mental health as an 'integral component of health and well-being' (WHO, 2022b). Elsewhere, they highlight four key points:

- Mental health is more than the absence of mental disorders.
- Mental health is an integral part of health; indeed there is no health without mental health.
- Mental health is determined by a range of socioeconomic, biological and environmental factors.
- Cost-effective public health and intersectoral strategies and interventions exist to promote, protect and restore mental health. (WHO, nd)

According to Kovacevic (2021), mental health has been largely overlooked for several reasons. Stigma is the one of the most pernicious obstacles to the diagnosis and treatment of mental illness. Another reason is the 'perception of mental health disorders as a "luxury good", as opposed to actual illnesses'. Additional reasons why mental health is overlooked relate to the piecemeal and outdated service models, including the provision of mental health services mainly in psychiatric hospitals and a chronic lack of preventative mental health services, as well as global policy development and long-standing workforce challenges.

Mental illness is a complex interaction between an individual's genetic, biological attributes and their economic and social environment. It is not an exact science and is approached from a range of standpoints. It can be difficult to separate fact from opinion. The past decade in the UK has been a time of momentous change around mental health. This subject, once considered taboo and discussed only in hushed tones, is now openly discussed and debated. Even so, it remains a controversial issue, surrounded by myths, stereotypes and stigma. The perception of mental illness has come a long way from its characterisation as an untreatable malady, with the unfortunate individual needing to be locked up in an asylum. While our understanding of mental health is evolving, there remain many gaps in knowledge and we still have a long way to go in understanding the brain. Fear is usually associated with the unknown, and this remains an issue when it comes to mental health.

This book is designed to be an accessible introduction to this contested policy area. It is primarily designed as a text for students of mental health but may also be useful to a range of other audiences, including social workers and nurses, or those with poor mental health and their families. The growth of multidisciplinary teams working in mental health has added impetus to the need for better understanding of key concepts and ideas. No single model is comprehensive enough to cover all aspects of mental illness. To reflect the varied terms used in discussions of mental health, we use terms such as mental illness, poor mental health, mental disorder and mental health interchangeably. This aims to avoid jargon and present information in a way that is straightforward and concise. Each chapter offers a bite-size introduction to key themes, though inevitably this is just the tip of the iceberg in terms of the knowledge and differing perspectives that exist. As the book is primarily aimed at a UK audience, and health and social care are fully devolved in the UK, when appropriate, reference is made to issues in Northern Ireland, Scotland and Wales. However, space does not allow for a full discussion of the extent to which the four nations of the UK have developed divergent legislation and policies.

This short guide has chapters covering the prevalence and cost of mental illness, mental health policy, issues of user involvement, the role of the voluntary, community and social enterprise (VCSE) sector, the social determinants of mental health, stigma and the portrayal of mental health in the media. We demonstrate that mental health policy is complex and does not sit in isolation from wider debates on funding of services, deprivation and the importance of early intervention. While the main focus is on the UK health and social care system, we also note some international trends and policy developments.

Chapter 1 focuses on the prevalence of mental illness and the models used to understand it. The extent of mental illness in the UK and internationally is described. In the UK one in four adults are likely to experience a mental health problem at some stage in their lifetime (Mind, 2016; Statistica, 2024). According to the Mental Health Foundation anxiety and depression are Britain's most common mental disorder. They estimate between 4 per cent and 10 per cent of people in England will experience depression in their lifetime (Mind, 2016). Can mental illness be cured? Can it be prevented? Can a person 'recover' from mental illness? This chapter briefly examines some of the most common mental illnesses, such as anxiety and depression, and other disorders such as post-traumatic stress disorder and bipolar disorder. It outlines the most common forms of treatment offered through the NHS, which include talking treatments and medication.

Chapter 2 explores the development of mental health policies in the UK. It outlines the move away from institutionalisation, or locking people up in asylums, towards community care. It covers legislation on detention and proposed amendments to the Mental Health Act 1983. It describes the multidisciplinary approach to care delivery, which involves the input of a range of health and social care professionals. It also discusses the development of forensic mental health services.

Chapter 3 sets out how mental health services are organised, looking first at the role of the state in service delivery for both adults and children and adolescents. The 'no wrong door' approach is described. Then the role of the VCSE sector in provision for mental health is considered, addressing barriers to involvement related to the statutory funding of VCSE organisations.

Chapter 4 discusses antipsychiatry and looks at the rise of the service user movement, exploring concepts such as empowerment, choice and control. It considers the concept of co-production and its implications. For some healthcare professionals, the idea of engaging with patients, and seeing providers and users of a service being mutually accountable, is controversial. The chapter considers the issue of power and notes that while it is neither possible nor desirable to share power equally in all situations, power dynamics can be reset. The significance of the idea of recovery and what this means to a range of stakeholders is outlined. The chapter also describes the establishment of recovery colleges, which incorporate co-production.

Chapter 5 examines the social determinants of mental illness, looking at issues such as poverty, gender, ethnicity and age. A person's mental health is shaped to a large extent by the social, economic and physical environment in which they live. Social inequalities are associated with increased risk of many common mental disorders. In some instances, disadvantage starts before birth and accumulates throughout the life course.

Chapter 6 turns to the key concept of stigma and outlines why this remains central to any understanding of mental illness. Negative societal responses to people with mental illness could be the single most important obstacle to addressing this health issue. The chapter reviews the nature of stigma and examines the different types of stigma, including public stigma, self-stigma and institutional stigma. Large-scale anti-stigma campaigns are discussed. The chapter also notes the importance of language in shaping norms and attitudes. It illustrates the ability of language to empower and, conversely, how words can marginalise and ostracise individuals.

Chapter 7 covers the relationship between the media and mental health. It examines the ways mental illness is frequently misrepresented and exaggerated, and how this reinforces stigma and social exclusion. There is an overwhelming emphasis on violence, with recovery and hope rarely afforded centre stage. Given the exponential rise in the use of social media, this chapter also reflects on how this influences mental health. The chapter sets out how social media can educate, enhance connection, increase self-esteem and encourage a sense of belonging. However, it is also associated with stress, pressure from comparing oneself to others, increased isolation and depression.

The Conclusion highlights the issues that have been identified and discussed throughout the book.

1

Mental health and mental illness

Introduction

Poor mental health has a significant impact on how people relate to others, make decisions and handle stress, and on their ability to achieve fulfilling lives. Mental health problems are complex biosocial processes that may develop over time. Defining what we mean by poor mental health and how we measure its prevalence are fraught with difficulties. Diagnostic labels are useful for clinical understanding and comparative research, but they cannot provide comprehensive insights into the nature and extent of mental disorders. This chapter provides an overview of the concept of mental health, the prevalence of mental illness, models of mental illness, the main types of disorder and the responses. It highlights some of the current and historical debates in this field and illustrates how diagnosis and treatments are informed by context and values.

The meaning of 'mental health'

Despite the increasing prominence of mental health as a policy issue, it remains poorly understood. The concept of mental health is complex, and there is a lack of consensus on definition. For example, the term 'poor mental health' is vague and often used interchangeably with, or as a euphemism for, 'mental illness', but their meanings are different. Mental health generally refers to a state of emotional, psychological and social wellbeing, while mental illnesses are diagnosed conditions that affect behaviours and quality of life. How mental illness should be defined and how disorders should be classified has been the subject of philosophical debates for decades. Arguments about what should and should not be included are often framed within wider debates about medicalisation, diagnosis, normality and clinical classification (Tse and Haslam, 2023).

Just as an individual may feel unwell but not have a recognised illness, people may experience poor mental health without having a mental illness. Good mental health does not mean feeling completely happy and relaxed all the time; rather, it is about maintaining a good quality of life and being equipped to cope with normal challenges and difficulties. As Kinsella and Kinsella (2015) explain, there are degrees of mental health. No one could really be described as having good mental health all the time. Many people will experience poor mental health in response to life events, such as bereavement, redundancy, physical illness and conflict. Others will experience mental health problems serious enough to warrant medical intervention. It is perfectly possible to have good mental health even with a diagnosis of a mental illness. Mental health issues exist on a continuum that covers a wide spectrum from psychosis through to more common experiences such as anxiety. The term has been defined in a multitude of ways depending on perspective, values, discipline and cultural norms. It is important to take this into account, as definitions have important implications for policy making and can also have legal ramifications.

The definition used by a psychiatrist will differ from one used by a service user or carer. In psychiatry, mental health issues are usually conceptualised in terms of illnesses with specific diagnostic guidelines, such as schizophrenia. Psychiatry has been criticised for being preoccupied only with mental illness. For some, mental disorders are conditions that can be consistently defined and have well-understood boundaries. Conversely, mental health appears to fall more into the realm of a subjective judgment. For example, mental illness can be defined as the presence of selected symptoms, but mental health is something more than the absence of symptoms. Definition of mental health as simply the absence of mental illness is too vague and closely associated with psychiatric value judgments, while definition based on wellbeing is too demanding and potentially oppressive

(Wren-Lewis and Alexandrova, 2021). Psychology focuses on the individual's behaviours and experiences rather than specific symptoms of a recognised disorder. For social work, the focus is on the social determinants of mental health, considering the relationship between an individual's experiences and the wider circumstances of their lives, such as poverty and social exclusion (Glasby and Tew, 2015).

The terminology associated with mental health and ill health can be confusing and contradictory, as terms are used by the general population and professionals in different ways. Warr (1987) notes that no universally accepted definition is available. Indeed, Shipman (1995, p 4) argues that mental health appears to be all things to all people. Herron and Mortimer (2000) emphasise that ideas about mental health are not fixed, but dynamic and subject to change in the light of new ideas or perspectives. This means that rather than seeing mental health as a discreet area of study, it is better understood as a multidisciplinary field in which ideas are often surrounded by controversy and debate. Mental ill health can be seen as a complex interaction between an individual's genetic, biological attributes and their economic and social environment.

Conflicting ideas about the causes and responses to poor mental health mean that there are different ways of understanding and framing the concept. Pilgrim (2017) contends that a recurring difficulty with trying to define mental health, or a mental disorder, is that it is almost impossible to clearly delineate between 'normal' and 'abnormal' states. Differences in values and norms vary over time and place, and this undermines attempts to formulate an agreed definition. What is considered 'normal' in one society may be viewed very differently in another. Mental health issues associated with subjective wellbeing are embroiled in historical relativism, value judgments and fantasy. For example, happiness is a core part of the American dream, with the pursuit of happiness a cherished right alongside life and liberty. Europeans have long been dubious about this fixation, and many dismiss it as ambiguous, superficial and banal. In addition, within a society, what is viewed as normal can change over time. Homosexuality was once viewed as a mental abnormality, but following extensive scientific research, the American Psychiatric Association (APA) declassified homosexuality as a mental condition. This led to significant shifts in the global mental health community. In 1990, the World Health Organization (WHO) removed homosexuality from the International Classification of Diseases (ICD). As a result of this decision, debates about homosexuality moved away from medicine and towards education, rights and discrimination. Consequently, cultural attitudes about homosexuality changed, and it was no longer considered an illness that needed to be cured or treated.

The WHO's definition of mental health is 'a state of well-being in which the individual realises his or her own abilities, can cope with the normal stresses of life, can work productively and fruitfully, and is able to make a contribution to his or her community' (WHO, 2014, p 1). This definition was widely welcomed as a move away from defining mental health as simply an absence of mental illness. However, while this definition is widely used, it has been the subject of considerable criticism and is no longer considered adequate. It describes a state of being that is static and impossibly idealistic. Wren-Lewis and Alexandrova (2021) contend that it is unrealistic for several reasons. First, it sets an incredibly high bar for achieving good mental health. Realising one's full potential, working productively and contributing to the community may be viewed as very demanding. Is it realistic to expect that individuals can fully realise these objectives? Many people who would describe themselves as well-adjusted and fully functioning may not actually live up to these standards. Second, it is unrealistic to suggest that people actually meet these standards. Third, it is framed in relation to functioning according to a set of norms, the normal stresses of life, productive work and contribution to society. But what about those who have a disability and are unable to participate in the paid labour market? Does this mean they cannot achieve a sense of wellbeing? If a person is unable to make an economic contribution, are they to be considered a burden, unlikely to achieve their potential?

Clearly, a definition of mental health is required that is dynamic, acknowledges the various challenges in the life cycle and places importance on the human capacity to cope with, and adapt to, new challenges. For example, for a healthy person who has lost their job in an environment where opportunities were scarce, having a state of wellbeing would be unexpected and unlikely. Over their life course, people who enjoy good mental health often experience sadness, anxiety and disappointment. This is perfectly normal and to be expected, yet ideas of mental health associated with happiness and the ability to control one's own destiny continue to persist. Wellbeing is subjective and may vary considerably between one person and the next. Furthermore, the focus in the WHO definition is firmly on the individual having responsibility for their own mental health, but mental health should be something that society collectively aims to achieve and promote.

Prevalence and impact of mental illness

No other condition comes close to mental illness in terms of prevalence, persistence and impact. It affects every aspect of life, including relationships, the ability to work, social connectedness and overall wellbeing. Across the globe, mental health has moved up the policy agenda, and a number of international organisations, such as the World Bank, the United Nations and the WHO, have attempted to set out the scale of the problem. For instance, in 2019, the WHO estimated that one in every eight people in the world live with a mental disorder, and most people do not have access to timely effective care (WHO, 2022c).

It is important to note, however, that there are significant limitations related to mental health data and a lack of reliable, robust information, which has resulted in knowledge gaps. Accurate measurement of mental health requires the development of indicators that capture the full spectrum of disease severity. Obtaining reliable and sustainable measures that allow for national and international comparison is complex and challenging. Additionally, the stigma associated with mental illnesses may deter many from disclosing an issue and seeking assistance. Assessing the treatments available is also fraught with difficulties due to the absence of clearly defined measures of treatment and inconsistent methodologies (Kilbourne et al, 2010). There is limited objective data across all four of the UK nations, with existing information often relying on self-reported indictors of wellbeing. According to the Royal College of Paediatrics and Child Health (nd), '[h]alf of mental health conditions in adults start before the age of 14, and 75% before the age of 24'. Furthermore, they note that in England, 'prevalence of all types of mental health conditions are increasing'.

Challenges of measurement

The Royal College of Paediatrics and Child Health suggest that mental health problems can be classified into four major groups:

- **Emotional disorders** (such as anxiety disorders, depressive disorders, mania and bipolar affective disorder)
- **Behavioural disorders** (characterised by repetitive and persistent patterns of disruptive and violent behaviour, in which the rights of others, and social norms, are violated)
- **Hyperactivity disorders** (characterised by inattention, impulsivity, and hyperactivity)
- **Others** (such as autistic spectrum disorder, tic disorders and eating disorders). (Royal College of Paediatrics and Child Health, nd, original emphasis)

According to the WHO, a mental health disorder is characterised by a clinically significant disturbance in an individual's cognition, emotional regulation or behaviour (WHO, 2022a). The ICD, which is produced by the WHO and periodically updated, is a comprehensive classification system for all physical and mental health diseases. It provides internationally recognised terminology that allows health professionals to frame their work and make diagnoses. It is also used by researchers to measure prevalence of mental illness and in planning for mental health provision. In January 2022, the 11th Revision (ICD-11) was implemented. The Diagnostic and Statistical Manual of Mental Disorders (DSM), published by the APA, also defines and classifies mental disorders. Both the ICD and the DSM are useful tools for categorising and understanding mental illnesses. They have evolved as knowledge and understanding has developed. For example, terminology and existing classifications are updated and new disorders are added over time.

However, the use of classification systems and categories for measuring complex mental illness has proved extremely contentious. In the literature, there is increasing recognition that these measurement systems do not reflect the complex interactions in systems involving biological, psychological and social elements (Fried et al, 2022). Also, importantly, the DSM and the ICD differ considerably in their conceptualization of some diagnoses (for example, diagnosis of post-traumatic stress disorder – PTSD). As well, there can be different measurement tools to diagnose the same disorder (for example, major depressive disorder; Fried et al, 2022). These differences mean it is difficult to be certain about the scale of mental illness, and as Vigo et al (2022) point out, the true global disease burden of mental illness remains unknown.

Critics of the classification systems also argue that attempts to apply precise scientific concepts to the human mind result in oversimplification and reductionism, which leads to misunderstanding. There is increasing dissatisfaction with long-standing conventional medical classifications such as the DSM. Richter and Dixon (2023) speculate that disputes may be related to the expansion of the domain of mental health.

Impact of mental health problems

There is a significant body of evidence indicating that mental health problems are a leading cause of disability worldwide and a significant risk factor for premature mortality (Patel et al, 2018; Arias et al, 2022). In the UK, mental health issues represent the largest cause of disability. In England, one in four adults suffers from at least one mental illness in any given year (NHS England, 2019). There is a substantial body of evidence that highlights the higher prevalence of mental health problems in Northern Ireland than elsewhere in the UK. The Northern Ireland Audit Office (2023) notes that estimates suggest mental illness is 25 per cent higher in Northern Ireland compared to England. These higher levels are associated with both poverty and the legacy of three decades of conflict (Northern Ireland Audit Office, 2023).

The Mental Health Foundation in England has published extensive research on the nature and extent of mental illnesses. Their work assesses the prevalence of mental health conditions and their direct and indirect costs. In 2022, they estimated the global cost of diagnosed mental health conditions and concluded:

- Mental health problems are one of the main causes of the overall disease burden worldwide.
- Untreated mental health problems account for 13% of the total global burden of disease. It is projected that by 2030 mental health problems (particularly depression) will be the leading cause of mortality and morbidity globally.
- Mental health and behavioural problems (such as depression, anxiety and drug use) are the primary drivers of disability worldwide, causing over 40 million years of disability in 20- to 29-year-olds.
- Major depression is thought to be the second leading cause of disability worldwide and a major contributor to the burden of suicide and ischemic heart disease. (Mental Health Foundation, nd)

The Lancet Commission on Global Mental Health and Sustainable Development, launched in 2018, outlined a proposal for 'scaling up' mental healthcare globally (Patel et al, 2018). The Commission highlighted that the inclusion of mental health in the United Nations Sustainable Development Goals provided an important opportunity to assess future directions for global mental health. The Commission, which included a team of 28 global experts, emphasised that every country in the world is facing a mental health crisis and all are failing to address it. According to these experts, despite advances in treatments and diagnosis, the burden of mental ill health is increasing everywhere. According to their report: 'The global burden of disease attributable to mental disorders has risen in all countries in the context of major demographic, environmental, and sociopolitical transitions' (Patel et al, 2018, p 1553). They recommend that mental health be given much higher priority, including parity with physical health services. Transformation of current systems requires an in-depth understanding of the scale of the impact of these disorders, including their distribution in the population, the health burden imposed and the broader health consequences. Mental illness exacts an enormous financial toll. In a 2023 report, the World Economic Forum indicates that a broadly defined set of mental health conditions could cost the world economy approximately US$6 trillion by 2030, low- and middle-income countries (LMICs) are likely to disproportionably bear the costs of these conditions (World Economic Forum, 2023).

In its largest review of mental health since the turn of the century, the WHO (2022c) note the high prevalence of mental health conditions in all countries and identify social and economic inequalities, public health emergencies, war and the climate crisis as significant global and structural threats to mental health. They also point out that in the first year of the COVID-19 pandemic, depression and anxiety increased by more than 25 per cent. They note too that suicide accounts for 1 in every 100 deaths and is a leading cause of adolescent death. The WHO report highlights that despite the scale of the problem, on average, governments spend just 2 per cent of their health budgets on mental healthcare, and LMICs spend just 1 per cent. Also roughly half the world's population lives in a country with one psychiatrist for 200,000 or more people. The report notes that child and adolescent mental health specialists are almost non-existent in many LMICs (WHO, 2022c). Consequently, most people living with mental illness do not get the appropriate care or support. In many LMICs, essential psychotropic drugs are often unavailable or unaffordable.

Prevalence inflation

The past ten years have been a period of considerable change in the area of mental health. There have been extensive efforts to raise public awareness about mental health problems and address long-standing taboos. Reported rates of mental illness have increased, and it has been suggested that this phenomenon may be partly explained by the concept of 'prevalence inflation' (Foulkes and Andrews, 2023) – that is, increased awareness may assist some people to recognise symptoms. In addition, some people may self-diagnose or demand a diagnoses, and this can lead to relabelling of milder forms of distress as mental health problems. Inflating diagnoses can mean resources are diverted away from small numbers of people who need them to large numbers of people who do not.

Mental health education campaigns may also, paradoxically, be contributing to the reported rise in mental health problems. Rather than rates of illnesses actually increasing, it has become more acceptable to report poor mental health. Alongside this, some mental health problems have acquired a cultural value, particularly on social media platforms. For example, depression may be viewed as cool. Social media platforms are being used not only to raise awareness on the issue, but also to alter the image of mental disorders. Many disorders – including anorexia nervosa, self-harm, depression and anxiety – are being glamourised and romanticised online. There is a need to ensure depictions are accurate and not subject to gloss and spin. Increased awareness can mean normal psychological experiences, such as mild anxiety or stress, become over-pathologised, resulting in milder forms of mental distress being reported as serious illnesses. This medicalisation of milder issues may not be helpful. For example, some people dealing with ordinary day-to-day stress are now self-diagnosing as having severe anxiety (Hasan et al, 2023). The false glamourisation of certain disorders has negative consequences, as it diminishes the seriousness of these illnesses (Williams, 2019). As well, the romanticising of certain conditions can further isolate people with other conditions, such as bipolar disorders or schizophrenia.

Risk of developing a mental disorder

Mental health is not experienced equally in the population. The prevalence of different mental disorders varies with age, gender, ethnicity and income group. Also, physical health problems significantly increase the risk of poor mental health and vice versa (Naylor et al, 2012). These inequalities relate not only to the prevalence of illness, but also to diagnosis and treatment (Bridges, 2014).

A significant body of evidence has shifted the concept of risk factor away from a fixed specific indicator towards a broader phenomenon that can change according to circumstances. Risk factors can reside within the individual or within the social structures that surround them. Genetic disposition, chronic illness, poverty, abuse, childhood adversity and trauma are generally recognised as important risk factors (Avison, 1992). They may also vary depending on the individual's age and stage of development.

In both men and women, anxiety disorders and depressive disorders are the most common mental problem. The Institute of Medicine (1994, p 168) suggests that there are five main risk factors associated with the development of depression:

- having a close biological relative with a mood disorder;
- the presence of a severe stressor, such as divorce, unemployment, chronic physical illness, trauma or inequality;
- having low self-esteem, low self-efficacy and a sense of hopelessness;
- being female;
- living in poverty.

Suicide accounts for 1 per cent of deaths worldwide, and is one of the leading causes of death in young people. It is estimated that there are 20 times as many suicide attempts as deaths by suicide. Suicide affects people, and their family and friends, worldwide, irrespective of age, country or context (WHO, 2022c).

According to the WHO (2022c), the main cause of 'years lived with disability' (YLDs) is mental disorders, with one in six YLDs attributable to mental disorders. Schizophrenia is a significant concern, as it is considered to cause the most impairment and occurs at a rate of 1 in 200 adults. People with severe mental health conditions, such as schizophrenia, die 15 to 20 years earlier on average compared to the general population, often from preventable diseases.

At any one time, a diverse set of individual, family, community and structural factors may combine to protect or undermine mental health. Although most people are resilient, people who are exposed to adverse circumstances – including poverty, violence, disability and inequality – are at higher risk. Protective and risk factors include individual psychological factors, such as emotional skills, and biological factors or genetics. Many of the protective and risk factors are influenced by changes in brain structure and function (WHO, 2022c).

UK suicide statistics

Suicide statistics in the UK jurisdictions show all deaths from intentional self-harm for people aged 10 or over. They also show deaths caused by injury or poisoning where the intent was undetermined; this covers people aged 15 and over. Figures are for deaths registered, not deaths occurring, in each calendar year, due to the time taken to complete an inquest, which can be months or even years.

England and Wales

In 2021, there were 5,583 suicides registered in England and Wales, equivalent to 10.7 deaths per 100,000 of the population (Office for National Statistics, 2022, np). This was statistically significantly higher than the 2020 rate of 10.0, but consistent with pre-COVID-19 rates in 2018 and 2019. The fall in the rate in 2020 was likely to have been driven by the decrease in male suicides at the start of the pandemic and delays in death registrations due to the pandemic. This is interpreted as evidence that the suicide rate did not increase due to the pandemic. Around three quarters (74 per cent) of people who died by suicide in 2021 were male, consistent with long-term trends. This was equivalent to 16.0 deaths per 100,000 of the population, compared to 5.5 for female suicides. In females, the age-specific suicide rate was highest among those aged 45–49, while for males it was highest among those aged 50–54 years. The largest increase in the period since 1981 (when the time series began) up to 2021 was for females aged 24 and under. Rates of suicide and self-harm in those aged 10–24 in England steadily increased in the decade up to 2021, and the steepest rise was among females, with this suicide rate doubling between 2011 and 2021. There has been speculation that factors including academic pressures, increasing social media use, family instability and drug dependence may be contributors, but evidence is limited.

Scotland

In 2021, there were 753 probable suicides in Scotland, a decrease of 6 per cent compared with the previous year and the lowest registered since 2017 (National Records of Scotland, 2022). Most of the decrease was due to a drop of 18 per cent in female suicides. The rate for males was consistent from 1994 to 2021, ranging from 2.6 to 3.6 times higher than females. Rates for suicide were highest among males aged 25–44 and 45–64, although suicides at age 25–44 fell in the decade up to 2021. The rate of suicide in the most deprived areas of Scotland was 2.9 times as high as in the least deprived – this gap was higher than the deprivation gap of 1.9 times for all causes of death.

Northern Ireland

Suicides in Northern Ireland are registered by the Northern Ireland Statistical Research Agency. In 2021, there were 237 suicide deaths (Northern Ireland Statistical Research Agency, 2022). This was the highest number since 2015 and represented an increase of 8.2 per cent from in 2020 (219 registered suicide deaths). Among those who died by suicide in 2021, 74.3 per cent were males and 25.7 per cent were females. The suicide death rate for both males and females was on an upward trajectory between 2019 and 2021. In the most deprived areas in Northern Ireland, the suicide rate was almost twice that in the least deprived areas (19.7 per 100,000 of the population and 10.8 per 100,000 of the population, respectively). In every year between 2001 and 2021, more than 70 per cent of suicide deaths in Northern

Ireland were male. In 2021, suicide deaths were highest for men aged 25–29 and 45–49, while for women the highest number of suicide deaths were for those aged 20–24. Overall in 2021, one in every three suicide deaths was someone under the age of 30, which was similar to previous years.

Models of mental health

Given that mental illness is one of the most controversial issues in the health sphere, it comes as no surprise that there are various models used to classify and shape our understanding of mental health. Experts from psychiatry, psychology, biology, philosophy, social policy and sociology have developed models to explain the essence of mental illness, interpret it and shape the response. Within the literature, there is fierce argument and debate about which are the most valid models and why. Those from different academic backgrounds and disciplines have disputed the advantages and disadvantages of alternative paradigms, approaches and models (Richter and Dixon, 2023). The various models usually have different goals and aims, and they propose solutions informed by their underpinning perspectives. This has led to debate about how symptoms and behaviours should be interpreted. Increasingly, there is an acceptance that mental health problems cannot be explained by adopting one approach, a position Kusch (2017) refers to as 'epistemic relativism'.

The idea of using a classification system to identify a poorly understood, contested health area has been met with robust resistance (Kinsella and Kinsella, 2015). Models are informed by underpinning perspectives, opinions and ideas, and they suggest different responses. Questions remain about fundamental issues such as what constitutes a mental illness or what mental health problems are. Theories about what is appropriate are still developing, and new communities are emerging. No single model is comprehensive; there is overlap of ideas, and each model has limitations. Based on extensive review of models of mental health problems, Richter and Dixon (2023) identify 34 models, which they group into five broad categories: biology, psychology, social, consumer, and cultural. They conclude that models are not clearly defined and individual models could be allocated to several of these categories.

The medical and biological models

Historically, mental health services were dominated by psychiatry and informed by the biological and medical models of disease. According to these models, exploring the anatomy of the brain is the best way to understand the origins of mental illness. The biological model is built on the assumption that mental illness can be explained by the brain and takes no account of other wider contextual issues. This model is underpinned by the medical model, which aims to diagnose and identify mental illness and prescribe a standardised treatment. The emphasis is on medication rather than therapy or counselling.

The complete focus on the biology of the brain proved fruitless and resulted in approaches which were both ill-informed and harmful. The most notorious surgical intervention was the lobotomy, pioneered in the 1930s by Egas Moniz. This involved severing the connection between the frontal lobe and other parts of the brain. In the US, the practice took on an even more macabre twist when Walter Freeman popularised the transorbital lobotomy, which involved severing connections in the brain with an ice-pick inserted through the eye sockets. In the United States, tens of thousands of these procedures were performed in the mid-1900s, often with devastating results. Following advances in knowledge, psychosurgeries are now relatively rare.

German psychiatrist Emil Kraepelin (1856–1926) was an influential figure who developed new ideas about the treatment of mental disorders. He proposed that there is a defined and discoverable number of medical disorders and that each of these is has a different cause and origin and follows a typical pattern. According to his analysis, in order to 'fix' people, it is first necessary to identify what is wrong with them, and the classification of a mental illness would provide the key to its biological origins. His ideas underpinned the disease model, which dominated psychiatry in the 20th century (Glasby and Tew, 2015).

According to Glasby and Tew (2015), the central tenets of the disease model are:

- Mental pathology is accompanied by physical pathology.
- Mental illness can be classified as different disorders, each of which has identifiable characteristics.
- Mental illness is biologically disadvantageous.
- The causes of physical and mental pathology in psychiatric illness are explicable in terms of physical illness.

The social model

The biological and medical models dominated debate on mental health until the emergence of the social model in the 1970s. The social model of mental health emphasises the social aspects that influence mental health disorders. Within this model, there is a wide range of differing views. These vary from the contention that social aspects are of singular importance to the suggestion that these are among several important variables.

Within the social model there are a number of influential theories, including social causationism, critical theory, social constructivism and labelling theory. Social causationism models stress the significance of social factors in isolation or in combination. This is illustrated in an influential study by Brown and Harris (1978) on working-class women in London. They found that women who had young children at home, lacked employment and had poorer social networks were more likely than other women to be depressed.

Pilgrim (2017) warns that emphasising the impact of social issues can result in social reductionism, which risks taking a simplistic view of a complex issue. Suggesting that everything is socially constructed ignores the psychological and biological realities. Focusing entirely on social factors could lead one to the conclusion that mental illness could be addressed by dealing with structural issues such as poverty, race, and gender.

Beresford et al (2010), in a study of service users' views on the social model of mental health, found that while the labelling and stigma that comes from the medical model of illness were major barriers to accessing timely, appropriate care, existing understandings of the social model were problematic for users of mental health services. A particular issue that created concerns for these service users was the concept of 'impairment' as part of the social model of disability. Some mental health service users were uncomfortable with this term, seeing it as negative and stigmatising. Beresford et al (2010) conclude that more thought is required about the usefulness of a social model of disability in this context. Another study found that while the social model was an empowering perspective for many with disabilities, others held the view that disability is completely due to social oppression, not individual impairment (Hogan, 2019).

Wallcraft and Hopper (2015) argue that a capabilities approach is the most appropriate way to challenge the dominance of the medical model. They claim that this can aid understanding of structural constraints and support a rights-based approach and recovery.

The psychosocial model

The psychosocial model aims to combine insights from both psychology and sociology to provide a more holistic understanding of mental health. By considering an individual's psychological make-up alongside the social environment, this model allows for a more comprehensive understanding of poor mental health and identification of appropriate treatment options. It is hoped that by realising the impact of these aspects on mental health, people can be empowered to better manage their mental health.

In terms of the relevance of social circumstances to wellbeing, establishing causal relationships is complex, as social context involves a multitude of factors. Nonetheless, one of the strongest predictors of life outcomes is education (Yu and Williams, 1999), and high level of education is associated with better mental health. People with higher levels of education have more choices and thus greater control over their lives and better security. Also, people who have completed higher education are liable to earn more throughout their lifetimes. Research evidence looking specifically at the association between education and depression has been inconsistent, but there is increasing support for a causation model. Kondirolli and Sunder (2022) found that people with higher levels of education suffer less severe symptoms of depression. They also found that the protective effects of education are higher for women and rural residents.

Forms of discrimination, such as racism, sexism and ageism, are also important social factors that affect mental health. Discrimination in all its guises can result in an erosion of self-confidence and create self-doubt, and the emotions associated with these experiences can have a negative impact on mental health. It has been shown, for instance, that racial trauma can affect one's ability to function effectively and maintain meaningful relationships (Williams et al, 2003).

Central tenets of the psychosocial model are:

- Mental ill health involves dysfunctional emotional, cognitive and behavioural processes (and the interrelationship between these).
- These may be understood as the consequence of difficult life circumstances.
- A person can experience difficulties when they rely on past beliefs, attitudes and coping mechanisms that are no longer appropriate to their current circumstances.
- Stressful personal relationships and wider societal factors – such as discrimination and lack of opportunities due to race, gender and social status – may increase the likelihood of experiencing mental ill health.
- Positive personal relationships and opportunities for social inclusion are crucial to long-term recovery.

The biopsychosocial model

In recent decades, there has been a move towards reconciling models to enable a more inclusive and holistic view of mental health. The biopsychosocial model was introduced by George Engel in 1977. He argued that for psychiatry to understand a person's medical condition, along with considering biological factors, it is important to look at psychological and social factors. This model takes account of a broader range of factors than the psychosocial model (Papadimitriou, 2017). Pilgrim (2002) explains that this model allows for a medical diagnosis, but values the individual and their social context over any medical category that may be applied to them.

The biopsychosocial model attempts to understand the relationship between:

- biology – physiological pathology;
- psychology – thoughts, emotions and behaviours, such as psychological distress, fear/avoidance beliefs, current coping methods and attributions;
- social context – socioeconomic, socio-environmental and cultural factors, such as work issues, family circumstances and personal financial circumstances.

This broad approach allows professionals to pinpoint key patterns in an individual's life, gain an insight into their family history and identify what factors impact on their quality of life. It is now widely accepted as the most appropriate approach to chronic pain. It recognises that pain is a psychophysiological behaviour pattern that cannot be categorised according to biological, psychological or social factors alone. The focus here is not about finding out what is 'wrong' with someone, but rather what happened to them. Treatments may include family therapy, cognitive behavioural therapy (CBT) and occupational therapies.

Common mental disorders

In this section, the most common mental disorders are described.

Anxiety disorders

Anxiety disorders are the most common of all mental disorders. The WHO (2022c) estimated that 301 million people worldwide

(4 per cent of the global population) were living with an anxiety disorder in 2019, including 58 million children and adolescents. Anxiety disorders are characterised by excessive fear and worry and related behavioural disturbances. People with these disorders may experience heart palpitations, sweating, nausea and trouble sleeping. Symptoms can be severe enough to result in significant distress or impairment in functioning. There are different kinds of anxiety disorder, including generalised anxiety disorder (characterised by excessive worry), panic disorder (characterised by panic attacks), social anxiety disorder (characterised by excessive fear and worry in social situations) and separation anxiety disorder (characterised by excessive fear or anxiety about separation from those individuals to whom the person has a deep emotional bond). There are a range of effective treatments for anxiety disorders, including psychological interventions to help people cope and, depending on the age of the person and the severity of the problem, medication. Barriers to care may include a lack of awareness and the inability to access treatment (Alonso et al, 2018).

Depression

Depression is a very common disorder that can be seriously debilitating. It is also very poorly understood. It was estimated that 280 million people worldwide were living with depression in 2019, including 23 million children and adolescents (based on data from WHO, 2022c). At some stage in their lives, everyone experiences feelings of low mood and despondency. However, depression is different from usual mood fluctuations and short-lived emotional responses to challenges in everyday life. During a depressive episode, or what professionals often term 'clinical depression', the person experiences depressed mood (feeling sad, irritable, empty) or a loss of pleasure or interest in activities for most of the day, nearly every day, for at least two weeks. Several other symptoms may also be present, including poor concentration, feelings of excessive guilt or low self-worth, hopelessness about the future, thoughts about dying or suicide, disrupted sleep, changes in appetite or weight and feeling especially tired or low in energy. People with depression have an increased risk of suicide. Like many other mental disorders, depression exists along a spectrum, and one person's experience may differ significantly from another's (Kinsella and Kinsella, 2015).

Bipolar disorder

Figures for 2019 revealed that 40 million people globally experienced bipolar disorder (WHO, 2022c). People with bipolar disorder experience alternating depressive episodes and periods of manic symptoms. Still sometimes referred to as manic depression, bipolar disorder belongs to the psychosis group of disorders. The popular view is that these are two states of mania. During a depressive episode, the person experiences depressed mood (feeling sad, irritable, empty) or a loss of pleasure or interest in activities for most of the day, nearly every day. Manic symptoms may include euphoria, irritability, increased activity or energy, increased talkativeness, racing thoughts, increased self-esteem, decreased need for sleep, distractibility and impulsive, reckless behaviour. Table 1.1 summarises the symptoms of manic and depressive episodes. People with bipolar disorder have an increased risk of suicide (Baldessarini, 2019). Yet effective treatment options exist, including psychoeducation, reduction of stress, strengthening of social functioning and medication.

PTSD

The prevalence of PTSD is high in conflict-affected settings (Charlson et al, 2019). An extensive study on the conflict in Northern Ireland and related trauma estimated that 8.8 per cent of the adult population met the criteria for PTSD at some point in their lives (CVS, 2011). PTSD may develop following exposure to an extremely threatening or horrific event or series of events. It is characterised by all of the following: re-experiencing the traumatic event or events in the present (through intrusive memories, flashbacks and nightmares); avoidance of thoughts and memories of the event(s) and avoidance of activities, situations or people reminiscent of the event(s); and persistent

Table 1.1: Symptoms of manic and depressive episodes

Symptoms of a manic episode	Symptoms of a depressive episode
Feeling very up, high, elated, extremely irritable, or touchy	Feeling very down or sad, or anxious
Feeling jumpy or wired, or being more active than usual	Feeling slowed down or restless
Racing thoughts	Trouble concentrating or making decisions
Decreased need for sleep	Trouble falling asleep, waking up too early, or sleeping too much
Talking fast about a lot of different things ('flight of ideas')	Talking very slowly, feeling unable to find anything to say, or forgetting a lot
Excessive appetite for food, drinking, sex, or other pleasurable activities	Lack of interest in almost all activities
Feeling able to do many things at once without getting tired	Unable to do even simple things
Feeling unusually important, talented, or powerful	Feeling hopeless or worthless, or thinking about death or suicide

Source: National Institute of Mental Health (nd)

perceptions of heightened current threat. These symptoms persist for at least several weeks and cause significant impairment in functioning. Effective psychological treatment exists including psychotherapy and medication (Watkins et al, 2018).

Schizophrenia

Schizophrenia is a debilitating mental health disorder that affects approximately 24 million people worldwide, or about 1 per cent of the global population (WHO, 2022c). Typically, individuals with schizophrenia have a life expectancy 10 to 20 years below that of the general population. It is a long-term, complicated mental health condition characterised by significant impairments in perception and changes in behaviour. It has a profound effect on not only the individuals affected and their families but also wider society. Symptoms may include persistent delusions, hallucinations, disorganised thinking, highly disorganised behaviour and extreme agitation. People with schizophrenia may experience persistent difficulties with their cognitive functioning. Effective treatment options include medication, psychoeducation, family interventions and psychosocial rehabilitation (Chien et al, 2013).

Eating disorders

In 2019, 14 million people worldwide experienced eating disorders, including almost 3 million children and adolescents (WHO, 2022c). Eating disorders are serious biologically influenced medical illnesses marked by severe disturbances to eating patterns. The most common are anorexia nervosa and bulimia nervosa: these involve abnormal eating and preoccupation with food as well as prominent body weight and shape concerns. The symptoms and behaviours result in significant risk or damage to health, significant distress and significant impairment of functioning. Anorexia nervosa often has its onset during adolescence or early adulthood, and it is associated with premature death due to medical complications or suicide. Individuals with bulimia nervosa are at a significantly increased risk of substance use, suicidality and health complications. Research suggests that involving families in treatment can be extremely effective in improving outcomes, particularly for adolescents (Erriu et al, 2020). Eating disorders can be treated successfully, and a range of treatment options exist, including psychotherapy, family-based treatment, cognitive-based therapy and medications.

Disruptive behaviour and dissocial disorders

It has been estimated that 40 million people worldwide, including children and adolescents, were living with conduct-dissocial disorder in 2019 (WHO, 2022c). This disorder, also known as conduct disorder, is one of two disruptive behaviour and dissocial disorders (the other is oppositional defiant disorder). Disruptive behaviour and dissocial disorders are characterised by persistent behavioural problems, such as being persistently defiant or disobedient and behaviours that repeatedly violate the basic rights of others or the major age-appropriate societal norms and laws. These disorders are typically first observed in childhood and can persist into adulthood. Unlike most other mental health conditions, with disruptive behavioural disorders, the individual's distress is focused outward rather than inward. Generally, these conduct behaviour issues are more common in males than females, with the exception of kleptomania (APA, 2018). Effective psychological treatments exist, often involving parents, caregivers and teachers; these treatments include cognitive problem-solving and social skills training.

Neurodevelopmental disorders

Neurodevelopmental disorders are behavioural and cognitive disorders that arise during the developmental period. They involve significant difficulties with acquisition and execution of specific intellectual, motor, language and social functions. Neurodevelopmental disorders include disorders of intellectual development, autism spectrum disorder and attention deficit hyperactivity disorder (ADHD). ADHD is characterised by a persistent pattern of inattention and/or hyperactivity-impulsivity that has a direct negative impact on academic, occupational and social functioning. Disorders of intellectual development are characterised by significant limitations in intellectual functioning and adaptive behaviour, which are associated with difficulties with everyday conceptual, social and practical skills performed in daily life. Autism spectrum disorder constitutes a diverse group of conditions characterised by some degree of difficulty with social communication and reciprocal social interaction, as well as persistent restricted, repetitive and inflexible patterns of behaviour, interests or activities. Effective treatment options exist, including psychosocial interventions, behavioural interventions, occupational therapy and speech therapy. For certain diagnoses and age groups, medication may also be considered.

Responses to mental illness

Mental disorders are a major health problem worldwide, and responses are often insufficient and inadequate. Almost every country in the world has failed to provide appropriate mental healthcare (Patel et al, 2023). Critical issues include the methods used to assess the nature of mental health, the dominance of biomedical approaches used to diagnose and treat mental illness, and workforce inadequacies. The gap between the need for treatment and its provision is wide all over the world, and when treatment is delivered, it is often poor quality. For example, only 29 per cent of people with psychosis and only 33 per cent of people with depression receive formal mental healthcare (WHO, 2023). In many LMICs, essential psychotropic drugs are often unavailable or unaffordable. Care in many countries is concentrated in long-term psychiatric hospitals (WHO, 2023). Research by Human Rights Watch (2019) has highlighted human rights abuses in these settings, where residents are often held against their will and may experience overcrowding, unsanitary conditions, obsolete medication and inadequate food. They also found that the number of professionals trained to provide treatment is wholly inadequate and service users are afforded few opportunities to express their preferences. The opportunity to participate in meaningful activities and support to develop and maintain personal relationships is also extremely limited.

The following discussion of treatments has been adapted from content on the Mind website (mind.org.uk).

Medications

While psychiatric medication eases the symptoms of mental health problems, it does not offer a cure. What it can do is allow a person whose symptoms are not severe to lead a normal life, or for someone with a severe condition, it can alleviate symptoms while the person receives additional help. Psychiatric medication can be prescribed to:

- treat a mental health problem;
- reduce the symptoms of a mental health problem;
- prevent a relapse of a mental health problem and its symptoms.

The following list shows the range of medications that can be prescribed:

- antidepressants (for depression and long-term anxiety);
- antipsychotics (for symptoms like hallucinations and delusions);
- mood stabilisers (for bipolar disorder, schizoaffective disorder and severe symptoms of some personality disorders);
- psychostimulants and stimulants (for ADHD and narcolepsy);
- anxiolytics (sedatives and anti-anxiety medications used to calm short-term anxiety);
- central nervous system depressants (to induce sleep);
- medications for substance misuse (to aid substance withdrawal and decrease substance misuse problems);
- cognitive enhancers (for Alzheimer's disease and other dementias, and cognitive impairment due to severe mental illness).

There may appear to be a great many medications for mental illnesses. However, they are all derived from groups of drugs. For example, Valium is a brand name for the generic drug diazepam, which is a type of benzodiazepine for the treatment of minor anxiety and insomnia. Some of the main groups of medications are described next, including the mental disorders they are used to treat.

Sedatives

Benzodiazepines are a type of sedative medication prescribed for severe anxiety or insomnia. They act on a natural chemical in the body called gamma-aminobutyric acid (GABA). GABA reduces activity in areas of the brain responsible for:

- reasoning;
- memory;

- emotions;
- essential functions, such as breathing.

Benzodiazepine drugs increase the effects of GABA on the brain and body to induce a feeling of relaxation and sleepiness, relax muscles and reduce anxiety.

Antidepressants

These are psychiatric drugs used to treat moderate or severe depression, or to help someone experiencing depression as part of another mental health disorder. They can also be used for:

- anxiety disorders and panic attacks;
- obsessive-compulsive disorder (OCD);
- phobias;
- bulimia nervosa;
- managing long-term pain.

In the UK, antidepressants are usually prescribed by general practitioners (GPs), but they can also be prescribed by psychiatrists, specialist nurse prescribers and specialist pharmacists. Although prescribed to treat the symptoms of depression, or another disorder, they do not deal with the causes. It is therefore likely that a GP will also prescribe 'talking therapy' (discussed later) to try to identify why the condition developed and help the person address it. Table 1.2 includes some of the more common medications for depression.

Antipsychotics

Antipsychotics are normally first prescribed by a psychiatrist to reduce the symptoms of the following disorders:

- psychosis
- schizophrenia (related to psychosis)
- schizoaffective disorder

Table 1.2: Common medications for depression

Generic drug	Effect of drug
Selective serotonin reuptake inhibitors (SSRIs) are the most widely prescribed type of antidepressant in the UK.	Serotonin is a neurotransmitter that sends signals between nerve cells. It has many functions, including regulating mood and sleep patterns. Low serotonin can cause depression, anxiety, insomnia and other mood disorders. SSRIs block the reuptake of serotonin into the nerve cell it was released from. This means it can act for longer in the body and brain.
Serotonin and noradrenaline reuptake inhibitors (SNRIs)	SNRIs work in a similar way to SSRIs, but they affect noradrenaline as well as serotonin uptake. Noradrenaline is a stress hormone affecting areas of the brain where reaction to stimuli is controlled. With adrenaline, it is responsible for the 'fight or flight' response, increasing the heart rate and causing increased blood supply to the muscles. These drugs are sometimes preferred when treating more severe depression and anxiety.
Norepinephrine-dopamine reuptake inhibitors (NDRIs)	NDRIs are similar to SSRIs and SNRIs in that they inhibit reuptake, but instead of inhibiting serotonin and noradrenaline, they inhibit the natural recycling process of norepinephrine and dopamine, increasing availability of these neurotransmitters in the brain to alleviate the symptoms of depression.
Tricyclics and tricyclic-related drugs	Tricyclics affect the uptake of noradrenaline and serotonin, but they also affect other chemicals in the body, so may be more likely to have side effects.
Monoamine oxidase inhibitors (MAOIs)	MAOIs work on an enzyme called monoamine oxidase to inhibit its breakdown of noradrenaline and serotonin. As with SNRIs, this means that noradrenaline and serotonin stay active for longer in the brain and body. MAOIs are only prescribed by a specialist, usually after other antidepressants have failed to be effective. This is because they can have dangerous interactions with certain foods and medications. Someone taking MAOIs will need to follow a strict diet and should check with a doctor or pharmacist before taking any new medication.

Source: adapted from Mind (nd-a)

Table 1.3: Categories of antipsychotics

First-generation antipsychotics – 'typical'	These fall into various chemical groups that act in a similar way and cause similar side effects. These include severe neuromuscular effects, though some will cause more severe movement disorders than others; drowsiness; and sexual side effects.
Second-generation antipsychotics – 'atypical'	Compared to first-generation antipsychotics, these cause less severe neuromuscular and sexual side effects, but they are more likely to cause serious metabolic side effects, such as rapid weight gain and changes to blood sugar levels.

Source: adapted from Mind (nd-b)

- some cases of severe anxiety
- bipolar disorder

Table 1.3 covers the difference between first-generation and second-generation antipsychotics.

These are just some of the drug treatments available for mental health disorders. They are prescribed to treat and ease the symptoms of disorders but they are not a cure. For example, while antidepressants may ease the symptoms of anxiety and panic attacks, they do not address the reason behind them. Therefore, they are often used in conjunction with other treatments, such as talking therapies, discussed next.

Talking therapies

The Improving Access to Psychological Therapies (IAPT) programme was launched in 2008 to improve delivery and access to therapies for depression and anxiety. The National Institute for Health and Care Excellence (NICE) has issued clinical guidelines recommending evidence-based psychological therapies as the first-choice intervention for depression and anxiety, including OCD. Studies have found that patients preferred psychotherapy to medication by a ratio of three to one, and waiting lists for talking therapies are extremely long (Clark,

2019). To help overcome this, NHS England trained more than 10,500 therapists to work in new psychological therapy services (Clark, 2019).

The programme is now known as NHS Talking Therapies, for anxiety and depression. To promote easy accessibility, the service can be accessed through self-referral or referral by GPs, community services and other mental or physical health services. The programme has been hailed as a success by the NHS, with 1.2 million people accessing services in 2021/22 (NHS England, nd-a). *The Five Year Forward View for Mental Health* (Mental Health Taskforce, 2016) and the *NHS Long Term Plan* (NHS, 2019) increased the target for people with anxiety and depression accessing the services to 1.88 million by 2023/24. The Nuffield Trust (2022) examined access to the programme over the period from 2011/12 to 2019/20 and found that the number of referrals starting treatment during this period had almost doubled. However, they concluded that the number beginning treatment would need to increase considerably for the 2023/24 target to be met.

NHS Talking Therapies for anxiety and depression provides interventions for adults and older adults. This can be a treatment, with or without medication, for anxiety and/or depression, or it can be provided alongside treatment for a long-term health condition. Treatment is provided for people with mild forms of the following mental health problems:

- agoraphobia
- body dysmorphic disorder (BDD)
- depression
- generalised anxiety disorder
- health anxiety (hypochondriasis)
- mixed depression and anxiety (the term for sub-syndromal depression and anxiety, rather than both depression and anxiety)
- obsessive-compulsive disorder (OCD)
- panic disorder
- Post-traumatic Stress Disorder (PTSD)
- social anxiety disorder
- specific phobias (such as heights, flying, spiders, etc). (NHS England, nd-a)

The types of talking therapy offered include the following NICE-recommended options:

- for depression – guided self-help based on CBT principles;
- for anxiety, including disorders such as panic disorder, phobias, OCD and generalised anxiety disorder (not advised for social anxiety disorder or PTSD) – guided self-help based on CBT principles;
- for PTSD – trauma-focused CBT;
- for social anxiety disorder – CBT. (NHS England, nd-a)

When patients begin treatment through the NHS Talking Therapies for anxiety and depression initiatives, they are clinically assessed and receive scores for their levels of anxiety and depression. Scores are monitored throughout treatment to measure progress. The recovery rate is the proportion of those who begin treatment as a clinical case and after treatment have a score below the clinical threshold.

Annual service outcomes for recovery are available on a public website (NHS Digital, nd-b). The recovery rate increased gradually between 2012/13 and 2018/19, with the target recovery rate of 50 per cent achieved in 2016/17. Since 2019/2022, the rate has fallen below target, to 49 per cent. NHS Digital notes that while the number of organisations that submit data for IAPT has not changed through the COVID-19 pandemic, there has been a significant change in the rate of recovery since the pre-COVID-19 period. Between February and April 2020, the number of referrals more than halved, likely due to the reduction in the number of patients presenting at GP surgeries during lockdown. The number of referrals starting treatment fell by 34 per cent over the same period. But since then both the number of referrals and the number starting treatment increased to levels slightly higher than before the pandemic (Nuffield Trust, 2022).

Principles of CBT and psychotherapy

Psychotherapy, or talking therapy, is a way to help people with a broad range of mental illnesses and emotional difficulties (APA, nd-b). Freud invented the psychoanalytic method, or the 'talking cure' (the presumption that talking has healing powers still fuels many psychotherapeutic practices). However, psychoanalysis and psychotherapy are different methods and have different goals. Psychoanalysis deals with the unconscious experiences that are beyond language and outside our awareness – the part of us that has been supressed by culture, social norms, rules and regulations. In contrast, psychotherapy deals with the 'ego' of active agency, whereby we make daily decisions. Psychotherapy works to restore a person's relationship with social norms and rules, while psychoanalysis works to strengthen their relationship with their own unconscious (Mental Health Digest, 2017).

CBT: This is a type of psychotherapy recommended by NICE for depression and all anxiety disorders. It helps people to identify and change thinking and behaviour patterns that are harmful or ineffective. CBT may be prescribed by a GP, or it can be accessed through self-referral. It is also offered by private counsellors at a cost in the region of £60 to £100 per session. CBT may be offered by the NHS as part of a 'stepped care' approach, meaning that if CBT is unsuccessful, other types of talking therapy or counselling can be offered.

CBT is a common treatment for a range of mental health problems, including depression, anxiety, panic attacks, stress, OCD, PTSD and phobias. It is based on the principle that thoughts, feelings, actions and physical feelings are all connected. How people think about situations can inform the way they feel and behave. If they think negatively, they will experience negative emotions, and this can become a negative cycle. For example, someone suffering from social anxiety may experience a panic attack in a social situation where they feel uncomfortable, and this reaction can add to and compound the negative associations they already have.

CBT combines two types of therapy to help deal with thoughts and behaviours: cognitive therapy examining thought processes and behaviour therapy examining subsequent actions. Unlike some talking therapies, CBT deals with the immediate problem rather than focusing on experiences from the past. The therapist works with the person to break down problems into separate parts – thoughts, feelings and actions. These areas are then analysed to determine whether they are unhelpful. The therapist helps the person work out how to change unhelpful thoughts and behaviours, and teaches the skills necessary to do so. The patient then applies these skills in their daily life and, at their next session, discusses how successful this has been. The eventual aim is to be able to apply these skills in daily life to help manage problems and stop them having a negative impact, even after the course of treatment finishes.

An advantage of CBT is that it can be completed in a relatively short period of time. Due to its highly structured nature, it can be provided in different formats, including in-person groups, online and self-help books. It teaches useful ongoing strategies, focusing on the person's capacity to change. It can be as effective as medicine for some mental health problems and may be helpful where medication alone has not worked. A disadvantage is that to get the most from the process, the person needs to commit to it, including attending sessions and applying learning between sessions. Other disadvantages are that it may not be suitable for people with complex mental health needs or learning difficulties, and it involves confronting emotions and anxieties without addressing wider problems that may be having an impact on the patient's wellbeing or the underlying causes of mental health conditions, such as childhood trauma.

Psychotherapy: Unlike CBT, psychotherapy examines the subconscious mind, looking at how childhood experiences are currently affecting the person's thinking, feelings, relationships and behaviour. Psychotherapy can also be delivered one-to-one or as couples therapy, family therapy or group therapy. Group therapy involves people with a common goal, and members can offer and receive support from the other group members, as well as practising new behaviours within a supportive environment.

It can be in the form of psychodynamic psychotherapy. The psychodynamic approach is derived from psychoanalysis, but focuses on immediate problems to try to provide a quicker solution. It stresses the importance of the unconscious and past experience in shaping current behaviour, based on the idea that behaviour and mental wellbeing are influenced by childhood experiences. The person works with the therapist to improve self-awareness and to change old patterns to gain more control of their life. Short-term psychodynamic therapy may be offered to people who have depression or anxiety plus a long-term mental health condition. It is offered as one-to-one therapy by the NHS, over around 16 sessions. Psychoanalysis is a more intensive form of psychodynamic therapy, with sessions often three or more times a week, provided for adults and older adults with severe mental health problems.

Psychological therapies are a key part of a new integrated offer for adults and older adults with severe mental health problems, such as psychosis, bipolar disorder, personality disorder and eating disorder. The NHS is seeking to increase availability of services for severe mental health problems as part of a wider transformation of mental health services.

Conclusion

Over the last five decades, there have been paradigm shifts in our understanding of and approaches to mental health. It is estimated that one in two people will suffer a mental disorder at some point in their lives (Queensland Brain Institute, 2023). Those affected may be treated by a mix of medicines, psychological therapies and social interventions. Mental health problems cannot be explained by a single approach, and there is continued debate about which model of mental health is the most valid. The existing models are based on different values and philosophies, and there is considerable overlap between them. There is increasing acceptance that user preferences should inform approaches and that their rights should be at the centre of collaborative initiatives.

Further reading

Augustus, J., Bold, J. and Williams, B. (2019) *An Introduction to Mental Health*, Los Angeles: Sage Publications Ltd.

2

Development of policy

Introduction

This chapter traces the progression of mental health services in the UK from the 13th century, when Bethlem Hospital housed people who had learning disabilities – deemed at the time to be 'insane' or 'lunatics' – and others who were simply poor and homeless. Reformers in the 1800s sought to address the dire conditions in mental asylums, bringing them to the attention of Parliament. Changing attitudes toward mental illness saw a new wave of asylums that were more progressive and offered therapeutic employment with a focus on recovery and rehabilitation. The establishment of the NHS in 1948 should have seen the integration of physical and mental health services; however, this was limited. The introduction of antipsychotic drugs in the 1950s made it easier to treat mental health patients outside of psychiatric hospitals. From 1961, government policy was to close the mental asylums and treat people with mental illness in general hospitals or integrate them into society; this process of deinstitutionalisation came to be known as 'care in the community' or 'community care'. Following several high-profile murders committed by psychiatric patients in the late 1990s, public concerns and media coverage shifted the policy focus from community care to public protection and risk management in the form of forensic mental health services legislation, which has been controversial. Mental health legislation in the devolved nations – Scotland, Wales and Northern Ireland – is briefly discussed before outlining the government framework for delivery of mental health care in the community through multidisciplinary teams (MDTs).

History of mental health services

This section describes the history of provision for people with mental health disorders and the early moves to reform institutionalised care.

Mental asylums

The term 'mental asylum' comes from the earliest religious institutions providing 'asylum' or refuge for the mentally ill. Before the introduction of those institutions, people with a mental illness or learning disability were cared for by their families or left destitute to beg for food and shelter. In England, psychiatric services date back to 1247, when the Priory of the New Order of Our Lady of Bethlehem was established in London (on the site where Liverpool Street station now stands) to provide shelter for the sick and infirm. From 1330, this became Bethlem Hospital, though it was commonly known as 'Bedlam' – a word still used to denote chaos or mayhem. Allegations in 1403 of malpractice and embezzlement of funds at Bethlem Hospital led to an investigation by a royal commission appointed by King Henry IV, which revealed that Bethlem Hospital was treating men with 'insanity' as well as physical illnesses (Killaspy, 2006).

At this time, mental illness was seen as a disease of the body rather than the mind. It was also believed that those with a mental illness were possessed by demons that could be purged by inducing recurrent vomiting and diarrhoea. As well as that, patients would have their heads shaved and be immersed in freezing baths. Unsurprisingly, these treatments, rather than offering a cure, often led to death. However, they were still universally accepted when Bethlem moved to a new premises at Moorfields in 1676, the UK's first hospital for the 'insane'.

By the 1700s, those with the financial means could send their 'mad' relatives to private institutions, which were virtually unregulated prisons in some cases. The poor, meanwhile, had to rely on local parishes, which sometimes provided charity-funded asylums, or else they ended up in workhouses or prisons. As Britain's only mental health facility, Bethlem had a long waiting list for admissions, and an increase in demand meant that the private 'madhouses' started to appear more often around London.

Reform

Around the beginning of the 1800s, reformers such as Samuel Tuke and Harriet Martineau spearheaded a change in attitudes toward mental healthcare. Concern began to grow about treatment, and in 1807 a House of Commons select committee set up to 'enquire into the state of lunatics' recommended the establishment of county asylums. Legislation in support of this included the County Asylums Act (Wynn's Act) 1808, which provided for 'the better care of and maintenance of lunatics', and the Lunacy Acts (Shaftesbury Acts) of 1845 'for the regulation of the care and treatment of lunatics' (Killaspy, 2006, p 247). Asylums were built on the outskirts of cities for patients living in surrounding rural areas. This heralded a change in emphasis from 'custody to cure', and Hanwell Asylum, established in 1832, was the first of a new wave of asylums. This institution took a progressive approach with therapeutic employment as part of patient care. Hanwell's extensive grounds were used for farming and recreation, and there was a bakery, a brewery and many other cottage industries to make the asylum as self-sufficient as possible.

By the early 1900s, public mental hospitals were overcrowded and underfunded, and patients were likely to spend most of their lives there, the emphasis being on care and control rather than cure. However, in the 1920s and 1930s, psychiatrists began to take a more interventionist approach, experimenting with new treatments for chronic mental conditions previously thought to be incurable, like schizophrenia. Working on the assumption that the conditions being treated had a physical cause, the treatments shown in Table 2.1 emerged.

Electroconvulsive therapy (ECT) is the only one of the therapies in Table 2.1 still used, to treat depression. In the 1960s, patients who had experienced ECT contributed to a movement questioning its use. It also emerged that it had been used on a disproportionate

Table 2.1: Controversial therapies

Treatment	Purpose
Insulin coma therapy	This therapy was used for the treatment of schizophrenia. Increasing doses of insulin were given until high enough to induce a coma. Introduced in 1927 in Vienna, by the 1940s it was being used in many US hospitals. It often resulted in heart failure or brain haemorrhage and death. Although questions were raised about whether it led to any long-term or lasting improvement, it continued to be widely used for schizophrenia throughout the 1940s and 1950s before being largely discredited in the 1960s and being discontinued.
Psychosurgery	This was a surgical procedure in which neural connections to and from the frontal lobes of the brain were severed. First performed in 1935, the theory of the Portuguese neurologist who invented it was that insanity was the result of fixed ideas supported by established neural pathways in the prefrontal lobes and disrupting these would relieve many of the symptoms of mental illness. The procedure was controversial with a low expectation of improvement. By the 1970s it had largely fallen out of use.
Lobotomy	A further development of psychosurgery was prefrontal lobotomy, although this was of questionable therapeutic value. It was believed by psychiatrists and patients' families that despite the often catastrophic consequences, a lobotomy would make the patient easier to manage and care for and was, therefore, a better option than lifelong institutionalisation. However, long-term studies of postoperative patients confirmed that the treatment was worse than the disease, and lobotomies were discontinued in most countries by the 1960s.
Electroconvulsive therapy	Developed in Italy in 1938, ECT was widely used across Europe. Views were positive in the early days of its use, although one long-term side effect was amnesia, and this could affect personal identity. Amnesia raised ethical questions around whether

Table 2.1: Controversial therapies (continued)

Treatment	Purpose
	patients, particularly those in psychiatric hospitals, could give informed consent for treatment. In the 1970s, a brief-pulse device with fewer side effects was introduced along with new conditions for informed consent plus supporting therapies and follow-up procedures. This therapy is still used though it remains controversial.

Source: adapted from Science Museum (2019)

number of women, people from Black and minority ethnic groups and people in LGBTQ+ groups. Negative representations in the media (for example, in the film *One Flew Over the Cuckoo's Nest*) also helped to turn both public and medical opinion against it. When it was reassessed in the 1970s, new conditions for informed consent were introduced along with supporting therapies and follow-up procedures. In the UK, the Royal College of Psychiatrists produced guidelines for its use and the Mental Health Act 1983 introduced a legal framework for the use of ECT on non-consenting patients. Modern ECT barely resembles the image in film and literature, although after years of clinical evidence and public scrutiny, its use remains controversial.

Deinstitutionalisation: from asylums to care in the community

From the establishment of the NHS in 1948, there has been disparity between physical and mental health services. This was partly due to mental illness being stigmatised, misunderstood and thought of as incurable, and the controversial history of mental health care. Parliamentary legislation used phrases such as 'lunacy' and 'mental deficiency' to describe patients.

In the early 1950s, advances were made in physical healthcare, but mental healthcare did not move forward and people were still detained in austere asylums. In 1954, Winston Churchill's government set up the Royal Commission on the Law Relating to Mental Illness and Mental Deficiency (chaired by Baron Percy of Newcastle and known as the 'Percy Commission') to review the detention of people with a mental illness and the existing legislative framework. The remit was to understand whether those with mental illness could be treated on a voluntary basis.

The Percy Commission's report in 1957 recommended that, where possible, people with 'mental disorders' should be treated in the community and not in large psychiatric institutions. The report stated that this would require expansion of community services and noted that barriers between the wider health system and mental health care should be broken down, with treatment for mental illness absorbed within the NHS. It also recommended that local authorities should provide accommodation to the mentally ill under the provisions of the National Health Service Act 1946 and the National Assistance Act 1948. However, integration of mental health services into the NHS was limited and closure of the asylums took many years, with mental health continuing to be mainly governed by legislation rather than policy.

It was not until 1959 that the first Mental Health Act was passed in England, replacing the Lunacy Act 1890. The Act defined mental illness as 'arrest or incomplete development of mind; psychopathic disorder; and any other disorder or disability of mind'. It provided the legislative framework for implementing the Percy Commission's recommendations. It removed the distinction between psychiatric and general hospitals to ensure that mentally ill patients could benefit from health and social services facilities, and it encouraged parity between mental and physical health care services. Section 6 of the Act placed a statutory duty on local authorities to provide aftercare to people with a mental disorder if they did not need inpatient care. Local authorities were required to provide and maintain residential homes for the care of these people as well as centres for training and ancillary or supplementary support services. Developments in service provision influenced policy trends. For example, the introduction of antipsychotic drugs in the 1950s meant that chronic psychological illnesses, such as schizophrenia, could be treated outside hospital (Prior, 1993). Until then, the preferred solution in most of the Western world, including Britain, had been institutionalisation to deal with the problems posed by serious mental illness.

In 1961, then Minister of Health Enoch Powell delivered his 'water tower' speech at the annual conference of the National Association for Mental Health (now the charity Mind), in which he announced a radical change in mental health policy that would eliminate most of the country's mental hospitals (Powell, 1961). The theme of the conference was providing an integrated service for mental disorders, which Powell stated 'could not possibly chime more perfectly with the aspirations to which the long-term planning for our hospital service is intended to give expression'. In relation to the asylums, he said:

> There they stand, isolated, majestic, imperious, brooded over by the gigantic water-tower and chimney combined, rising unmistakable and daunting out of the countryside – the asylums which our forefathers built with such immense solidity to express the notions of their day. Do not for a moment underestimate their powers of resistance to our assault. […] We have to strive to alter our whole mentality about hospitals and about mental hospitals especially. (Powell, 1961)

The Mental Health Act 1959 led to the closing down of asylums and psychiatric care being absorbed into the wider hospital system, with mental health services 'thereafter developed against a background of serial reorganisations of the NHS and local government' (Turner et al, 2015, p 602). The process began in 1962 when Powell launched the NHS Hospital Plan for England and Wales, which set out the aim to develop a programme of hospital building and put the focus on community care and the role of primary care professionals (see HoC, 1962).

Support for the closure of asylums was not universal. Sociologist Erving Goffman argued that although the situation in asylums was 'deplorable', they existed because there was a desire and need for what they offered, and he called for 'sober-minded forbearance rather than reform'. He wrote:

> Mental hospitals are not found in our society because supervisors, psychiatrists, and attendants want jobs; mental hospitals are found because there is a market for them. If the mental hospitals in a given region were emptied and closed down today, tomorrow relatives, police and judges would raise a clamor for new ones; and these true clients of the mental hospital would demand an institution to satisfy their needs. (Goffman, 1961, p 384)

Goffman's theory of 'total institution' focused on the relationship between 'guard' and 'captor'. While he focused on asylums, his theory can also be applied to other institutional settings, such as prisons and hospital wards. Goffman demonstrated the way in which 'inmates' and staff interacted to strip patients of their identity in order to re-socialise them into the rules and routines of the institution – in other words, 'institutionalising' them.

The closure of asylums was due to moral conscience and a growing awareness of human rights issues, although there was also a belief that it would save money. Scull claims that the policy of deinstitutionalisation was pursued over decades even as it became clear that community care 'was simply a figment of politicians' imaginations, a phrase that sought to obscure the fact that there was little in the way of community to which most mental health patients could return and still less in the way of care' (2021, p 307). He disputes the argument that advances in pharmaceutical interventions for mental illness in the 1950s contributed to the closure of asylums, noting that the greatest number of discharges from asylums took place from the 1970s, when there were no breakthroughs in psychopharmacology. Scull argues that it was policy rather than availability of drugs that informed deinstitutionalisation.

UK government white papers HMSO June 1971 and HMSO October 1975 proposed abolishing the mental hospitals, with services being delivered in general hospitals, supported by general practitioners and social services. The white papers suggested that mental illness was not only an issue for hospital services, but also a social issue. Inpatient and outpatient facilities in general hospitals became part of psychiatric care and a resource for assessment and treatment. There was also a commitment to community-based services, including supported housing, day care services and community-based mental health nurses and social workers. Early critics of care in the community cited examples of those discharged from mental hospitals becoming homeless, to show that it had failed. However, long-term studies found that outcomes were good for the majority of those who had previously lived in asylums, even those with complex issues. They increased their social networks, gained independent living skills, improved their quality of life and did not require readmission to hospital (Killaspy, 2006).

The optimism of the initial period of deinstitutionalisation was replaced during the 1980s and 1990s by wider societal concerns about pressure on services and a focus on individuals in crisis, which marginalised user/survivor voices (Cummins, 2018). High-profile murders committed by mental health patients living in the community led to a focus on forensic mental health services designed to protect the public.

Forensic mental health services

Forensic mental health services specialise in the assessment, treatment and management of people with mental health needs who have previously undergone or are currently undergoing legal or court proceedings. Some are managed by forensic mental health services because they are considered a risk to themselves or others. Services encompass high-, medium- and low-security provision, or provision in the community, with the level determined by the risk the person is assessed as posing. It has been argued that in practice patients end up in forensic mental health services 'when the nature of their offending, or apprehension about their behaviour, is such as to overwhelm the tolerance or confidence of professionals in general mental health services' (Mullen, 2000, p 307).

Until 1997, the policy focus on improving care for those with severe mental illness was mainly driven by public concern following media reporting of serious incidents involving psychiatric patients (Turner et al, 2015). This included the high-profile case of Christopher Clunis, a man with a diagnosis of schizophrenia, who murdered Jonathan Zito in an unprovoked attack at Finsbury Park station in London in 1992. With the controversial care in the community approach, the focus became one of risk assessment and risk management. It was thought that general hospitals would not have the skills or experience to manage patients with challenging or violent behaviour, and there was a culture of blame in which medical professionals feared they could be accused of failing to protect the public.

Legislation on detention of mental health patients

Legislation on the detention of mental health patients is provided in England and Wales by the Mental Health Act 1983 (amended in 2007). A Code of Practice was published in 2015 (Code of Practice: Mental Health Act 1983, January 2015) providing statutory guidance for registered medical practitioners, approved clinicians, managers and staff providers on how they should carry out their functions under this Act. The 1983 Act defines mental disorder as a disorder or disability of the mind. Changes to the Act in 2007 included: a widening of the definition of mental disorder; the initiation of mental health advocacy for some detained patients; the expansion of the range of professional roles involved in the process; and the introduction of new provisions for supervised treatment in the community following discharge from hospital, known as community treatment orders (CTOs). In 2013, the House of Commons Health Select Committee scrutinised the 2007 amendments (House of Commons Health Committee, 2013) and covers areas of concern including:

- rising rates of detention under the Mental Health Act;
- variation in the use of CTOs;
- problems with independent advocacy for supporting patients;

- over-representation of Black and minority ethnic groups among those detained.

In 2013, the Upper Tribunal (Administrative Appeals Chamber) considered the interaction between the Mental Health Act 1983 and the Mental Capacity Act 2005 in the *AM v SLAM NHS Foundation Trust* case. The tribunal found the following:

1. The tribunal should first determine whether a patient has the capacity to consent to arrangements in Section 131 of the Mental Health Act if they lack capacity.
2. Alternatives the tribunal should consider are whether the hospital could rely on provisions of the Mental Capacity Act to lawfully assess or treat the patient. This involves two issues:
   a) Are they eligible for Deprivation of Liberty Safeguards (DoLS) under the Mental Capacity Act? If they object, they are then ineligible for DoLS?
   b) Would DoLS be required? (DoLS are necessary when there is a risk that objectively amounts to a deprivation of liberty.)
3. The tribunal should take the least restrictive approach in compliance with Article 5 of the European Convention on Human Rights. The Mental Health Act must be applied such that detention in hospital is 'necessary' and cannot be achieved by less restrictive measures.

This case emphasises the need to consider Mental Capacity Act alternatives and the least restrictive approach when determining whether detention under the Mental Health Act is warranted.

Continuing concern prompted the government to appoint an independent review body in October 2017, chaired by consultant psychiatrist Professor Sir Simon Wessely to review the use of the Mental Health Act and what could be improved. The resulting report, published in December 2018, concluded that the Act needed serious reform. It stated that rates of detention under the Act were rising, with disproportionate numbers of Black and minority ethnic groups being detained, and that processes were out of step with a modern mental health care system. Wessely, while acknowledging the level of public fear following Zito's murder, believed that media coverage and public discourse at the time of the murder was a driver of the perceived need for reform of the 1983 Act and had brought about the 2007 amendment. The mental health care system was seen to have failed to adequately manage the risk posed to the public from people with a diagnosed mental illness. However, it was Wessely's view that acts of violence by psychosis patients are rare, and this was reiterated recently by Scull, who argues that the media coverage induced a moral panic causing a 'distortion of policy that found legislative recognition in the new category of "Dangerously Severe Personality Disorder" (DSPD) in the 2007 Mental Health Act' (Scull, 2021, p 310).

The independent review (Department of Health and Social Care, 2018) made 154 recommendations to reform law and practice. These focused on human rights and patient choice and autonomy, and included proposals for: advance documents to allow people to set out their wishes about their care and treatment; providing them with skilled advocates; patients being able to choose a family member or friend as a 'nominated person' to be involved in decisions on the use of compulsory powers; an increase in the scope of tribunals to review detention and any concerns around care; and a statutory right to a care and treatment plan. The government's response in December 2018 was to take forward only two of the recommendations: the proposals for advance choice documents and nominated persons.

The Queen's Speech (highlighting the government's priorities for the coming parliamentary year) in October 2019 announced the plan to reform the Mental Health Act when parliamentary time allowed. Detailed proposals were delayed in 2020 by the COVID-19 pandemic, but were published in a government white paper in January 2021. The white paper contained proposals to modernise mental health legislation to ensure care and treatment promotes recovery. Recommendations included raising the threshold for compulsory detention, limiting the use of the Mental Health Act for people with a learning disability and people with autism, and a range of measures to improve the experience of people from Black and minority ethnic groups. The overall aim of the reforms was to bring legislation in line with modern mental health care, allowing patients more involvement in decisions about their care and treatment. A consultation on the white paper proposals took place from January to April 2021, and this found broad support for the proposals.

The Queen's Speech in May 2022 announced draft legislation to reform the Mental Health Act 1983, describing it as a 'once in a generation reform to bring the Mental Health Act into the 21st century and give people greater control over their treatment and receive the dignity and respect they deserve'. On 27 June 2022, the Secretary of State for Health and Social Care, Sajid Javid, introduced the draft Mental Health Bill to 'modernise legislation' and 'make sure that it is fit for the future'.

The draft Bill underwent pre-legislative scrutiny before being introduced in Parliament. The Joint Committee on the Draft Mental Health Bill published its report on 19 January 2023. The Joint Committee supported reform but wanted the government to strengthen the Bill to address rising detention rates and racial inequalities. Among the Joint Committee's recommendations were introduction of a new statutory mental health commissioner role, the abolition of CTOs and the introduction of statutory advance choice documents for patients to make choices about their future care and treatment. Measures were also proposed to improve the experience of people from Black and minority ethnic groups. Reform was also proposed for those with serious mental illness who are in contact with the criminal justice system, focusing on rehabilitation and a reduction in reoffending. There were also proposals aiming to stop people with autism and/or learning disabilities from being detained. At the end of March 2021, there were 2,035 people with learning disabilities and/or autism detained in inpatient units, and of these, 735 had been detained for five years or more (NHS Digital, 2021). This was in line with the national plan *Building the Right Support* (Department of Health and Social Care, 2015) and the *NHS Long Term Plan* (NHS, 2019) to develop community services and close inpatient facilities for those with a learning disability and/or autism who display challenging behaviour.

Amendments to the Mental Health Act 1983 contained in the Bill included:

- redefining 'mental disorder' so that autistic people and those with a learning disability cannot be treated under Section 3 of the Act without a coexisting psychiatric disorder;
- raising the threshold for detention and more frequent review of the need for detention;
- replacing the 'nearest relative' with a 'nominated person' of the patient's choice as someone who can make decisions when necessary;
- expanding access to advocacy services;
- removing prisons and police cells as places of safety;
- for patients in the criminal justice system, introducing a 'supervised discharge' and a statutory 28-day limit for transfer from prison to a hospital.

Currently an 'approved mental health professional' decides whether to use the Mental Health Act or the Mental Capacity Act to detain people. The independent review and government white paper (HM Government, 2021b) proposed to change this so that decision makers would use the DoLS or Liberty Protection Safeguards rather than the Mental Health Act if a patient either does not object to detention and treatment or lacks the mental capacity to object. Where a person objects to detention and treatment, the Mental Health Act should be used. However, following public consultation, the government decided not to include these proposals in the Mental Health Bill.

The King's Speech on 7 November 2023 did not refer to the Mental Health Bill. This meant that the Bill would not be passed by the then Conservative government before the general election (which was later set to take place in July 2024), despite reforms to the Mental Health Act (1983) being a key commitment in the Conservative Party manifestos in 2017 and 2019. Dr Sarah Hughes, Chief Executive of Mind, said the chance had been missed to address the deep racial injustices in the use of the Act, with Black people being four times more likely to be detained. Hughes claimed this was further evidence of the lack of regard the then UK government had for mental health, especially given reports of unsafe mental healthcare in the UK (Mind, 2023).

UK devolved nations

Since 1999, health and social care has been a devolved matter in Scotland, Wales and Northern Ireland. Health and social care policy and legislation in each jurisdiction is summarised next.

Scotland

One in three people in Scotland are affected by mental ill health in any one year and as such it is stated to be a major priority by the Scottish Government (2022a).

The main mental health legislation in Scotland is the Mental Health (Care and Treatment) (Scotland) Act 2003, as amended by the Mental Health (Scotland) Act 2015. The 2003 Act applies to people who have a mental illness, a personality disorder or a learning disability. It places duties on local councils to provide them with care and support services, and it aims to develop community-based mental health services and involve service users and unpaid carers in decisions concerning treatment. The Act allows for compulsory measures only when there is a significant risk to the patient or others. The Act was amended in 2015, and changes came into force in 2017. These included allowing service users quick and easy access to treatment and measures around 'named persons' and advance statements and advocacy rights. It also introduced a 'victim notification scheme for victims of mentally disordered offenders'.

A review of mental health law in Scotland was undertaken with a public consultation. Its aim was to ensure that mental health is given parity with physical health. The final report was published in 2022 (Scottish Mental Health Law Review, 2022).

Scotland's suicide prevention action plan, *Every Life Matters* (Scottish Government, 2018), set out a target to reduce the rate of suicide by 20 per cent by 2022 (from a 2017 baseline). A National Suicide Prevention Leadership Group was established to support delivery of local prevention plans. Its fourth annual report (Scottish Government, 2022b) indicated that the effectiveness of the approach was recognised by the WHO. The group no longer exists having taken forward the development of Scotland's new suicide prevention strategy, *Creating Hope Together* (Scottish Government, 2022c).

Wales

Mental health legislation in Wales is provided by the Mental Health Act 1983, the Mental Capacity Act 2005 and the Mental Health (Wales) Measure 2010. The Mental Health Act and the Mental Capacity Act apply to both England and Wales, and these were discussed earlier in relation to England.

The Mental Health (Wales) Measure 2010 places new legal duties on local health boards and local authorities for the assessment and treatment of mental health problems. It also improves access to independent mental health advocacy services.

Northern Ireland

Northern Ireland has had an integrated health and social care model for over three decades. Despite this, mental health has been regarded as the 'Cinderella' of health and social care, with the emphasis being on acute hospital services for people experiencing mental illness (O'Neill et al, 2019). In 2002, the Department of Health, Social Services and Public Safety (now the Department of Health) initiated a review of the law, policy and provisions for people with mental ill health or a learning disability (see Department of Health (Northern Ireland), nd). The review was known as the 'Bamford Review' in recognition of the contribution of the late Professor Bamford, who was Chair of the steering committee.

In 2019, despite there being strong evidence that Northern Ireland had high levels of mental illness and suicide rates that were the highest in the UK and throughout Ireland, it had never had a mental health strategy (O'Neill et al, 2019). Mental health service reform was still guided by the 2002 Bamford Review, although the direction of travel in healthcare policies and strategies demonstrated an evolution towards the 'health and wellbeing' of the general population (O'Neill et al, 2019). However, following lobbying by the mental health sector, the *Mental Health Strategy 2021–2031* was published in June 2021 (Department of Health (Northern Ireland), 2021) and a mental health champion was appointed in September of the same year to further the mental health agenda in Northern Ireland.

The Bamford Review had proposed a single legislative framework for Northern Ireland, recommending the 'fusion' of mental health law (primarily concerned with the reduction of risk to the patient and others) and mental capacity law (designed to empower people over 16 to make decisions for themselves wherever possible and to protect people who lacked mental capacity to make decisions about their care). This finally happened when the Mental Capacity Act (Northern Ireland) 2016 received Royal Assent on 9 May that year. This was the first time mental capacity had been defined through legislation in Northern Ireland, and it is also widely recognised as the first time in the world that mental health law and mental capacity law have been incorporated into the same piece of legislation (Betts and Thompson, 2017). An 2016 academic paper describes it in its title as 'No longer "anomalous, confusing and unjust"' (Harper et al, 2016).

A key recommendation from the Bamford Review was to move away from hospital-based care to community care for those with a mental illness or a learning disability. Historically in Northern Ireland, as part of the proposed expansion of health services in 1950, it was estimated that there was a need for a further 1,500 beds in mental hospitals and 1,000 beds 'in a colony for "persons requiring special care"' (Prior, 1993, p 327). The planned 'colony', meant for people with a learning disability, was not realised until the end of 1960, when 600 patients were living in the new 'colony' in Muckamore Abbey Hospital, outside Antrim. Sadly the 'special care' the patients received there resulted in the largest major safeguarding issue the NHS has ever faced, and a public inquiry was announced in September 2021 into allegations of abuse at the hospital.

The Chair of the public inquiry, Tom Kark QC, in his opening statement at the start of proceedings on Monday 6 June 2022, said: 'What happened at Muckamore Abbey hospital has been referred to as a scandal and without predetermining any issue it is quite obvious that bad practices were allowed to persist at the hospital to the terrible detriment of a number of patients' (quoted in BBC News, 2022). Staff were alleged to have carried out physical and mental abuse as well as 'wilful neglect' of vulnerable patients. After viewing 300,000 hours of CCTV footage from inside the hospital, 34 people were arrested, 8 were charged and a further 70 staff were suspended as a precaution (BBC News, 2022). Some of the patients at the hospital were nonverbal, so unable to report what was happening, while others were vulnerable and not believed.

Community care

As discussed earlier, deinstitutionalisation and care in the community has been one of the most controversial policy shifts of the late 20th century, due to not only the media-induced 'moral panic' involving several acts of violence but also the fact that the National Health Service and Community Care Act 1990 passed responsibility for care to local authorities without providing them with adequate resources. Scull (2021) argues that when the political and moral focus turned to maligning mental institutions, this deflected from meaningful assessment of the community care alternatives being prepared for people being discharged from institutions. This put a tremendous strain on families, who were unwilling to complain, creating a false belief that they were able to cope. Research has shown that 'the burden on relatives and the community was rarely negligible, and in some cases, it was intolerable' (Wing and Brown, 1970, cited in Scull, 2021, p 311).

There had been an assumption that community care would be cheaper than institutional care (Bergmark, 2017), although studies found that for someone with high levels of need, the cost of providing support in the community could be higher than the cost of hospital care (Killaspy, 2006; Scull, 2021). Older age and high levels of disability were associated with higher costs, and costs were also felt by families providing unpaid care, often with little or no support from social services (Killaspy, 2006; Scull 2021).

In the 21st century in the UK, there has been a commitment to parity of esteem for mental health and physical health (NHS, 2014). It is argued, however, that there is not a single accepted measure for the concept of parity of esteem. It can be measured according to equal funding, equal access to services or equal life expectancy (Garratt and Laing, 2022). In relation to the gap in life expectancy between those with a severe mental illness and the general population, which has been estimated at 15–20 years, the government committed to ensuring that by 2020/21, 280,000 adults with a severe mental illness would receive an annual health check (Garratt and Laing, 2022). An evaluation found that data from NHS Digital suggested the target had not been met and was not on target to be met prior to the COVID-19 pandemic (House of Commons Health and Social Care Committee, 2021).

Ever-expanding definitions have led to the emergence of new manifestations of mental ill health, and models of care need to adapt and expand to accommodate these. The *NHS Long Term Plan* (NHS, 2019) has had to address developments such as internet addiction, online gambling and gaming addiction among children and young people. In October 2019, NHS England announced the opening of the National Centre for Behavioural Addictions to support children and young people seriously addicted to online computer games. The centre also supports internet addiction and is located alongside the National Problem Gambling Clinic, which offers a gambling addiction service for young people.

There is a realisation in recent policy developments that mental health issues are not solely the domain of health and social care. The focus on the concept of wellbeing acknowledges that mental and physical health is impacted by social, economic and community status, and by issues related to housing, education, employment, social interaction and loneliness. The continuing development of MDTs aims to address social as well as mental and physical health issues.

Multidisciplinary approach to care delivery

The rationale for MDTs developed with community-based care. MDTs are made up of professionals across primary care, community care and social care, who work together to plan a patient's care. Depending on the needs of the patient, a mental health MDT may include a consultant psychiatrist, a psychologist, a psychiatric community nurse, a social worker and possibly a physiotherapist and an occupational therapist. Teams can also include voluntary care professionals. Actions within these teams can range from one professional calling on other staff for support or input to multiple professionals sharing responsibility for a single patient.

Research has shown that the most effective MDTs are those with an identified care coordinator. This can be a facilitator or manager, or one of the team members involved in delivering care. The care coordinator role can be fundamental to the success of MDTs. To carry out the role effectively, the care coordinator's background or professional skill set is less important than their 'people' skills (The King's Fund, 2013, p 16). Tracey et al argue that health and social care are not working effectively together as 'existing models are too rigid, linear, discouraging of innovation and ill-equipped to deal with what they now face' (2023, p 16). They also point out the challenges of bringing together a workforce with different culturally distinct services and pay scales (Tracey et al, 2023) – this is not a new observation, as the fact that most MDT members are employed by the NHS but social workers who are part of MDTs are employed by local authorities was raised as an issue two decades ago (Carpenter et al, 2003). A recent study found that there is a lack of clear rationale for the social worker role in mental health services in England and Wales (Tucker et al, 2022).

As part of the NHS New Models of Care programme launched in 2015, local partnerships were selected to be 'vanguards' that rapidly implement innovative service change. A report in 2017 found that where NHS vanguard sites included mental health professionals in care models, early results were promising – for example, when mental health expertise was included in integrated care teams, it was reported by other team members that this was 'highly valuable in improving the support delivered to people with complex and ongoing care needs' (Naylor et al, 2017, p 3). The overall assessment, however, was that opportunities to improve mental health care through integrated approaches had not been fully realised and insufficient priority was given to mental health in developing the new models of care. This was not consistent with the commitment in *The Five Year Forward View for Mental Health* (Mental Health Taskforce, 2016) to parity of esteem between mental and physical health. Naylor et al (2017) argue that this must be a priority if progress is to be made.

Conclusion

In the UK, austerity and associated policies have combined to increase the overall burden of mental distress and marginalisation. Demands on mental health services are increasing – this was anticipated following the social isolation of lockdowns during the COVID-19 pandemic and later with the cost-of-living crisis.

The UK government has made a commitment to parity of esteem for mental and physical healthcare. Healthcare policies and strategies cite aspirations to deliver undefined concepts such as 'wellbeing', 'person-centred care', 'co-production' and the inclusion of 'lived experience' in planning and delivering mental healthcare services. However, without clear definitions and measurable outcomes, how will we know if parity has been reached and what it will look like?

The challenge faced by health and social care throughout the UK is mainly focused on acute services with overcrowded emergency departments in hospitals, lengthy waiting lists for initial consultant appointments and treatment, and a shortage of healthcare staff. The healthcare crisis has led to the introduction of the Major Conditions Strategy (Department of Health and Social Care, 2023). The aim is to prioritise and alleviate pressure on the healthcare system. It is also intended to reduce ill health related to economic inactivity. While mental illness and dementia are included in the six areas this Strategy is intended to address, it nonetheless comes instead of a stand-alone mental health strategy for England, which had been promised for a decade.

If a comparison is drawn between mental health services now and in the past when patients were virtually imprisoned in austere asylums, then services have come a long way. Alternatively, if a comparison is drawn between mental health services and acute services, the picture is less positive, as parity of esteem is still a long way off.

Further reading

Ikkos, G. and Bouras, N. (eds) (2021) *Mind, State and Society: Social History of Psychiatry and Mental Health in Britain 1960–2010*, Cambridge: Cambridge University Press [Open access]. doi: 10.1017/9781911623793

3

Organisation of mental health services

Introduction

This chapter looks at how mental health services are delivered in the UK. This includes a discussion of the role of both the state and the voluntary, community and social enterprise (VCSE) sector. Separate services have been developed for different groups (for example, children and young people), and these are accessed in various settings and delivered by a range of providers. Community mental health services now play a crucial role in the UK, offering services such as psychological therapies, trauma-informed care, support for self-harm and help for suicide ideation. New models of care have been built around integration and mutidisciplinary working. Community services have been modernised to offer support through whole-person, whole-population approaches. Integrated care systems (ICSs) have been developed to transform, improve and expand community mental health services. New strategies emphasising the importance of choice, control and empowerment have been published in all regions of the UK.

In response to the marginalisation of people with mental health difficulties, the WHO (2021a) and the OECD (2021) have called for a more integrated, holistic, person-centred and recovery-oriented approach to the care of people with mental health difficulties to be embedded into the design and delivery of services. Ensuring that services respect the preferences of individuals is far from straightforward, however. It involves systemic shifts in structures, practices and beliefs alongside sustainable funding and ongoing political support (Sharek et al, 2002).

Role of the state in service delivery

The WHO (2022c) reports that globally one in eight people live with a mental health disorder, the most common disorders being anxiety and depression. They argue that while well-defined policies and plans for mental health provision are important, 'simply having a plan in place is not enough to meet mental health care needs: plans need to comply with human rights instruments, be fully resourced and implemented, and regularly monitored and evaluated'; they also say that 'within mental health budgets, community-based mental health care is consistently underfunded' (WHO, 2022c, pp 54 and xv).

In the UK in 2011, the Coalition Government introduced its mental health strategy, *No Health Without Mental Health* (HM Government, 2011). This set out the ambition to mainstream mental health and establish parity of esteem between services for mental and physical health. It set out six key objectives:

(i) More people will have good mental health. [...] Fewer people will develop mental health problems. [...]

(ii) More people with mental health problems will recover [... and they will have] stronger social relationships, a greater sense of purpose, the skills they need for living and working, improved chances in education, better employment rates and a suitable and stable place to live.

(iii) More people with mental health problems will have good physical health. Fewer ... will die prematurely. [...]

(iv) More people will have a positive experience of care and support [... and this] should offer access to timely, evidence-based interventions and approaches that give people the greatest choice and control over their own lives [...]

(v) Fewer people will suffer avoidable harm [... and they] should have confidence that the services they use are of the highest quality and at least as safe as any other public service.

(vi) Fewer people will experience stigma and discrimination. Public understanding of mental health will improve. (HM Government, 2011, p 6)

In 2015, evidence showed that many people did not know where to go for support if they experienced a mental health crisis (All Party Parliamentary Group on Mental Health, 2015). A mental health crisis was described as having suicidal behaviour or intention, panic attacks and extreme anxiety, episodes of psychosis and behaviour that seems out of control to the person and others around them. However, emergency mental healthcare was found to be the starkest example of the lack of parity between physical and mental health (All Party Parliamentary Group on Mental Health, 2015).

There was a lack of clear referral routes and no single point of access. A freedom of information request by mental health charity Mind (2015) revealed that local authorities were spending on average only 1.36 per cent of their public health budget on mental health. Health and wellbeing boards – charged with bringing together those responsible for commissioning NHS, social care, public health and VCSE sector services locally – were failing to prioritise mental health services. A key reason was the failure of health and wellbeing boards to collect adequate data on the level of mental health need in their area to inform public health strategies. The data that existed was often outdated and incomplete.

In 2015, although it was estimated that one in four people in the UK were affected by mental health problems, accounting for 23 per cent of total ill health, only 13 per cent of the NHS budget was allocated to mental health (All Party Parliamentary Group, 2015). By 2021/22, the £12 billion NHS spend on mental health services had fallen to the equivalent of around 9 per cent of the NHS budget, even though between 2016/17 and 2021/22, the number of people in contact with mental health services increased from 3.6 million to 4.5 million (National Audit Office, 2023). Some key facts from the National Audit Office's (2023) *Progress in Improving Mental Health Services in England* report are shown in Figure 3.1.

The commitment in the *NHS Long Term Plan* (NHS, 2019) to boost mental health services spending by £2.3 billion a year should enable

Figure 3.1: Key facts related to NHS England services

Key facts

4.5mn

number of people in
contact with NHS-funded
mental health services
during 2021-22

£12.0bn

NHS spend on mental
health services in 2021-22,
equivalent to around 9%
of the NHS budget

4.9 times

People with severe mental
illness more likely to die
prematurety than the general
population during 2018-2020

**22%
(24,000)**
increase in NHS mental health workforce between 2016-17
and 2021-22

44%
increase in referrals to NHS mental health services
between 2016-17 and 2021-22, from 4.4 million in
2016-17 to 6.4 million in 2021-22

8 million
NHS England estimate of the number of people with mental
health needs not in contact with NHS mental health services,
as of 2021

1.2 million
estimated number of people on the waiting list for
community-based NHS mental health services at the end
of June 2022

26%
estimated proportion of 17- to 19-year-olds with a probable
mental disorder in 2022, increasing from 10% in 2017

17%
proportion of NHS mental health funding spent on
non-NHS providers, including independent and voluntary
sector providers, in 2021-22

61%
for July to September 2022, proportion of referrals to
talking therapy services excluded from calculation of
waiting time standards

Source: National Audit Office (2023)

around 4.5 million adults and over 700,000 young people to access
mental health services.

In addition, in 2022, a press release from the Department of Health
and Social Care (2022) announced a capital investment of £150 million

for mental health crisis response and emergency care up to April 2025. This includes £7 million for the procurement of around a hundred mental health ambulances to either take specialist staff directly to the patient to provide support at the scene or to transfer them to an appropriate place of care. The remaining £143 million is to provide new, or refurbish existing, mental health response infrastructure. This includes 20 new or improved health-based places of safety for people detained by the police.

The aim of the investment is to allow patients experiencing a mental health crisis to receive care and support outside of A&E departments, helping to reduce pressures on the NHS. It will provide tailored emergency care in the community, including 150 new projects to support mental health crisis response and urgent healthcare. The funding also covers step-down services (providing support during transition from hospital to community based care) and crisis line upgrades, including improvements to NHS 111 (the digital triage service in England) and crisis phone lines. As well, it covers improvements to health-based places of safety (places with mental healthcare staff based in the community). These include crisis cafes, safe havens and sanctuaries, and provide a safe and supportive space in the community and an alternative to A&E. Community-based support in crisis houses can provide more intensive support, and this can include overnight stays where necessary.

Child and adolescent mental health services

Of the 3,256,695 people known to have been in contact with secondary mental health services, learning disability services and autism services at some point in 2021/22, 992,647 were under 18 years of age (NHS Digital, 2022a).

The Mental Health of Children and Young People Survey found that for children aged 7–16, rates of mental disorder rose from one in nine (12.1 per cent) in 2017 to one in six (16.7 per cent) in 2020 (NHS Digital 2022b). Rates remained stable up to 2022. However, there was a slightly different pattern for young people aged 17–19 years: rates of probable mental disorder rose from one in ten

Figure 3.2: Mental disorder in children and young people in England, 2017–22

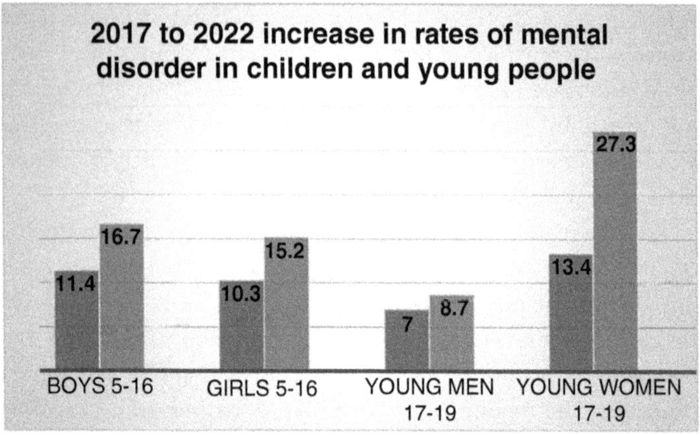

Source: NHS Digital (2022b)

(10.1 per cent) in 2017 to one in six (17.7 per cent) in 2020 and were stable in 2020 and 2021, but then increased to one in four (25.7 per cent) in 2022. A series of surveys showed that four in ten children and over half of young people surveyed reported a deterioration in their mental health between 2017 and 2022 (see Figure 3.2). While these statistics will have been affected by the COVID-19 pandemic, it is impossible to quantify the impact (NHS Digital, 2022b). Data for 2022 also showed that among 7- to 16-year-olds, 28.3 per cent of those with a probable mental disorder had self-harmed at some time in their life, compared with 2.5 per cent of those who were unlikely to have a mental disorder (NHS Digital, 2022b).

Among children aged 7–10 years, boys were almost twice as likely as girls to have a probable mental disorder in 2022 (19.7 per cent of boys compared with 10.5 per cent of girls). This was reversed among older age groups, as among those aged 17–19, girls were more likely than boys to have a probable mental health disorder (33.1 per cent and 18.7 per cent, respectively) (NHS Digital, 2022b).

Children with special educational needs and disabilities (SEND) were more likely to have a probable mental health disorder than those without SEND (56.7 per cent compared to 12.5 per cent) in 2021 (no breakdown was provided for 2022; Baker and Kirk-Wade, 2024).

NHS child and adolescent mental health services (CAMHS) operate throughout the UK, assessing and treating children and young people up to the age of 18 for emotional, behavioural and mental health difficulties. (Children and young people's mental health services is a new term for CAMHS that is being used in England.) Care teams include nurses, therapists, psychologists, child and adolescent psychiatrists, support workers and social workers. CAMHS can also refer to community-based services that provide a range of services for mental illness or addiction concerns. Children and young people can be referred for a CAMHS assessment by a general practitioner (GP), a school, a social worker or a health visitor.

Families and carers of children and young people with mental health problems have made it clear that they need timely access to evidence-based quality care in the right place and more services provided in the community. They find it unacceptable that children and young people have to travel long distances for care or be placed inappropriately on paediatric acute wards or adult psychiatric wards. Some have complained that they struggle to access inpatient services at all. To address this, NHS England are taking steps to improve community services (NHS England, 2019).

In January 2017, a package of reforms to improve mental health services in England was announced (see Garratt et al, 2022), and this referred to the importance of early intervention for children and young people. The package included:

- offering mental health first aid training to every secondary school in the country and trailing ways to strengthen links between schools and local mental health services;
- tasking the Care Quality Commission to lead a major thematic review of CAMHS;
- publishing a new green paper on transforming mental health services for children and young people in schools and universities, taking families into consideration as well;

- supporting NHS England's commitment to eliminate inappropriate inpatient placements for children and young people by 2021. (Garratt et al, 2022)

In 2016, the government introduced waiting time standards for access to eating disorder services for children and young people. By 2020/21, a target of 95 per cent of children and young people were to have received treatment within a week of referral for urgent cases and within four weeks for routine cases. However, targets had not been met during the quarter ending December 2023, with 64 per cent of urgent cases being seen within one week, and 79 per cent of routine cases within four weeks (Baker and Kirk-Wade, 2024).

Some services, such as talking therapies and early-intervention psychosis services, have waiting time targets, but many services have no official data on how long patients wait between referral and treatment. Improving Access to Psychological Therapies outcomes by age and gender for 2021/22 showed that younger people were less likely to experience recovery than older people, with the 50 per cent recovery target for those under 25 not reached (Baker and Kirk-Wade, 2024).

The Mental Health of Children and Young People Survey in England in 2022 found that 11- to 16-year-olds with a probable mental health disorder were less likely to feel safe at school and less likely to report enjoyment in learning or having a friend they could turn to for support. School-based counselling has shown positive outcomes. Unlike CAMHS, where there is a mental health diagnosis, children do not present with specific mental health disorders. However, some children prefer to be referred to services outside the school environment due to the perception that school services may be less discreet and anxiety about their peers knowing they are seeking help (NHS Digital, 2022b).

Outside the statutory sector, the VCSE sector offers counselling services for children and young people. One study found that clinical outcomes for services offered by the VCSE were comparable to those for statutory services, including services in schools. They were also perceived to be accessible and able to reach marginalised groups that had not accessed other services (Duncan et al, 2021).

CAMHS in Northern Ireland

As noted in Chapter 1, there are especially high levels of mental illness in Northern Ireland, and this is the case for children and young people as well as adults. It is estimated that at any one time around 45,000 children and young people in Northern Ireland have a mental health problem (Betts and Thompson, 2017). A survey by the Prince's Trust in 2018 of 2,000 16- to 25-year-olds in Northern Ireland found that 44 per cent of young people had experienced a mental health problem and that 68 per cent always or often felt stressed, 60 per cent always or often felt anxious and 33 per cent always or often felt hopeless (Prince's Trust, 2018).

A 2019 report on mental health services (O'Neill et al, 2019) found that CAMHS was still shaped by the Bamford Review of Mental Health and Learning Disability, launched in 2002, which reported that CAMHS was under-resourced, fragmented and lacked strategic vision (see Chapter 2).

In July 2012, a 'preferred' model for the organisation and delivery of CAMHS was published, and this introduced a stepped care model with five levels of support: prevention; early intervention; specialist intervention services; crisis intervention; and inpatient and regional specialist services (Department of Health, Social Services and Public Safety (Northern Ireland), 2012a). However, the stepped care approach has received some criticism from practitioners and service users based on children and young people being passed from service to service; this has happened because individual services struggle due to insufficient resources to cope with demand.

An evaluation by the Education and Training Inspectorate (2018) looking at emotional wellbeing and support in schools found that schools were struggling to cope with demand for counselling services. Although schools could access support services through the Education Authority and healthcare services, the evaluation found that some schools had to use their own resources to access support in urgent cases. It also highlighted reports of counselling services and other interventions being too short to be effective.

Also according to the evaluation, the five most common areas that impacted on pupils' health and wellbeing were anxiety, stress, anger, relationships and home life. Bereavement, suicidal ideation, identifying as transgender, body image issues, self-harm and social deprivation were also identified as important. Anxiety was the biggest issue relating to schoolwork, friendships and family issues. Social media was an issue where it involved inappropriate sharing of information that led to bullying and social isolation (Education and Training Inspectorate, 2018).

The *Still Waiting* review by the Northern Ireland Commissioner for Children and Young People (NICCY) found that the core budget for children and young people had not kept pace with recommendations for service reform. There was underinvestment, and some funding was allocated to services that were not based on known mental health needs. This meant that there was a mixed experience in terms of availability, accessibility and quality of services (NICCY, 2018).

Responding to NICCY's review, the Royal College of Paediatrics and Child Health (2020) said that with less stigma around mental health services, demand had increased and services had failed to keep pace with this. This lack of support could have a lasting influence on young people's lives in relation to, for example, employment prospects and risk of drug and alcohol misuse. They called for policy makers to ensure that those working with children and young people were trained to identify signs of mental health issues so that early intervention could take place. They noted that children should be able to access mental health services at any time, whether through the education system, primary care or child health services. However, for this to happen, they argued, services would need to be integrated and properly funded (Royal College of Paediatrics and Child Health, 2018).

Community Mental Health Framework for Adults and Older Adults

The WHO recognises the importance of delivering community mental health services, and they have published guidance (WHO,

Table 3.1: Foundations for change

Frameworks	Commitment	Finance	Competencies
• Laws, plans and policies • Research and information	• Political will • Public interest • Community action	• Domestic finance • External investment	• Healthcare workforce • Community providers • Self-care

Source: WHO (2022c)

2021) on community mental health services globally, covering crisis services, community outreach, peer support, hospital-based services and supported living services. The WHO's *World Mental Health Report* further highlights the need for community-based mental health services (WHO, 2022c; see Table 3.1).

In England, the *Community Mental Health Framework for Adults and Older Adults* (NHS England, 2019) replaced the Care Programme Approach (CPA), which had been in effect for almost three decades. The CPA had a central role in supporting people with severe mental illness in the community, based on care planning and case management, but it had not been updated for 15 years. Community mental health policy and practices had changed significantly over this time, and there was new legislation in the form of the Care Act 2014. Prior to the *NHS Long Term Plan* (NHS, 2019), core community mental health services had received negligible increases in funding for many years, and a range of stakeholders had raised the concern that the CPA was acting as a major barrier to the provision of the high-quality, flexible and personalised care service users needed (NHS England, 2022).

The Framework sets out the vision for community mental healthcare for adults with serious mental illness, and the intention is to provide coherence for local services' approaches to care coordination, care planning and case management. NHS England's CPA position statement (Version 2.0) stated that one of the purposes of the Framework is to 'enable services to shift away from an inequitable, rigid and arbitrary CPA classification and bring up the standard of care towards **a minimum universal standard**' (NHS England, 2022, p 2, original emphasis).

The new approach involves providing intervention-based care with a named key worker. There is to be a clearer multidisciplinary team (MDT) approach when assessing needs, and reliance on care coordinators should be reduced. Drawing on new roles – including lived experience roles – it envisages co-produced, holistic, personalised care for those with severe mental health problems living in the community. There is also to be more support for and involvement of carers, including improved communication and the opportunity for family members to contribute to care and support planning. The aim is to produce a more accessible, responsive and flexible system that can address fluctuations in the individual's condition over time. This offers a personalised approach, based on high-quality assessment. The level of planning and coordination of care can be tailored and amended, depending on:

- the complexity of the person's needs and circumstances at a given time;
- what matters to the person and the choices they make;
- the views of carers and family members;
- professional judgement.

The Framework is based on five broad principles:

(i) A shift from generic care co-ordination to **meaningful intervention-based care** … which helps people recover and stay well ….

(ii) **A named key worker for all service users with a clearer** … **MDT** approach to both assess and meet the needs of service users … drawing on new roles including lived experience roles.

(iii) **High-quality co-produced, holistic, personalised care and support planning for people with severe mental health problems living in the community:** a live and dynamic process facilitated by the use of digital shared care records and integration with other relevant care planning processes … with service users actively co-producing brief and relevant care plans with staff, and with active input from non-NHS partners where appropriate including social care (to ensure Care Act compliance), housing, public health and the voluntary, community and social enterprise … sector.

(iv) **Better support for and involvement of carers** as a means to provide safer and more effective care. This includes improved communication, services proactively seeking carers' and family members' contributions to care and support planning, and organisational and system commitments to supporting carers in line with national best practice.

(v) **A more accessible, responsive and flexible system** in which approaches are tailored to the health, care, life needs, and circumstances of an individual, their carer(s) and family members, services' abilities and approaches to engaging an individual, and the complexity and severity of the individual's condition(s) which may fluctuate over time. (NHS England, 2022, pp 3–4, original emphasis)

The 'no wrong door' approach

In terms of making mental health services more accessible, the 'no wrong door' approach is being adopted in some public services in the UK. This approach to public services originated in America when the Affordable Care Act, formally known as the Patient Protection and Affordable Care Act, became law in March 2010. One provision of the Affordable Care Act, known as the No Wrong Door Policy, was to enable people to complete a single application to allow the government to determine what health and social services programmes they were eligible for. The initial implementation aimed to break down silos across health departments, but advances in technology made it possible to apply the approach across different government services. Now in the US, a single application can determine if someone is eligible to enrol in government programmes such as Medicaid, the Children's Health

Insurance Programme, Temporary Assistance for Needy Families and community-based services.

In the UK, the approach is being applied as a people-centred solution to stop individuals falling through gaps in public service provision. It was first used by North Yorkshire County Council (now North Yorkshire Council) for children's social care, and an evaluation of that work indicated that the no wrong door model had made substantial progress in achieving its aims (Lushey et al, 2017).

In 2022, looking to the future with this model, the NHS Confederation in partnership with the Centre for Mental Health published a vision of what mental health services, autism and learning disabilities could look like in ten years' time (Bell and Pollard, 2022). Their vision for 2032 includes some of the reasons why mental health services in England must change (see Box 3.1).

Box 3.1: Reasons mental health, autism and learning disability services must change

The following findings were reported in 2022:

- The economic and social cost of mental health problems in 2019/20 was **£119 billion**.
- **About 10 million** more people, 1.5 million of them under 18, will need extra support for their mental health because of COVID-19.
- **Only 1/4 to 1/3** of people with a mental health difficulty receive treatment for it.
- **1 in 6 children** had a mental health difficulty compared with 1 in 10 in 2004 and 1 in 9 in 2017.
- **Higher rates** of most common mental health difficulties are in women and girls than men and boys.
- **3x more likely** to find a mental health difficulty in children with a learning disability.
- **More than 75 per cent** of autistic people sought support for their mental health in last five years.

- **More than 2,000** people with autism and people with a learning disability are in a mental health hospital, the vast majority under the Mental Health Act.
- **An average of 15–20 years** shorter life expectancy in people with learning disabilities and people with long-term mental health problems compared with the general population.

Source: Bell and Pollard (2022, p 10, emphasis added)

The report identifies ten interconnecting themes that underpin the vision for a reform of services by 2032 (outlined in Table 3.2) and three key requirements for the vision for mental health, autism and learning disability to become a reality: 'sustained and sufficient investment'; 'effective long-term workforce development and planning'; and 'a deep commitment to large-scale reform, innovation and change' (Bell and Pollard, 2022, p 7).

The cornerstone for the vision is that by 2032 there must be no wrong door for anyone seeking support for mental health, autism and learning disability. People should be able to present at any point in the system – from pharmacies to advisory services, the criminal justice system and primary care – and get the right support (Pollard and Bell, 2022).

The Royal College of Psychiatrists in Scotland called on the 2021–26 Scottish Parliament to use the no wrong door approach in addressing mental health issues in Scotland (Royal College of Psychiatrists, nd). Their policy priorities were:

- By 2022, a multidisciplinary mental health workforce plan, alongside the refresh of the mental health strategy, that provides the staffing needed to provide care at the point of need
- A guarantee mental health receives its share of funding to meet people's need post Covid, and that we move towards 10% of frontline health spend to meet the mental health needs of all Scots

Table 3.2: Interconnecting themes for the NHS Confederation and Centre for Mental Health's vision for mental health, autism and learning disability in 2032

Theme	Description
1. Prevention	Locally and nationally, government and public services will take a systematic 'population health' approach to reducing the social and economic risk factors for poor mental health.
2. Early intervention	Early intervention will be the norm, with support front-loaded at an early stage. Services will meet people where they are at, including online, at school, and in community spaces where they feel comfortable.
3. Access to quality, compassionate care	There will be no wrong door. People will be able to present at any point in the system – from pharmacies, advisory services and community groups to education, social services, the criminal justice system and primary care – and get the right support.
4. Seeing the bigger picture	People will get support with what matters most to them and services will help people with money, work and housing – with a package of support that is not limited to 'healthcare' per se.
5. Whole-person care	Services will support people with their physical and mental health and social needs together. Services will treat people as whole person, being mindful and respectful of their needs, assets, wishes and goals.
6. Equality focus	Services will be proactive in addressing structural inequalities and injustices.
7. Co-production	Coproduction as an equal partnership will be the norm in the design, development, and delivery of services.
8. Autonomy, human rights and community support	Service users will be reaping the benefits of a major investment in community support. As changes to the Mental Health Act will have channelled investment away from institutional and inpatient services, comprehensive support in the community will have risen to support people's needs.
9. A stronger workforce	There is a thriving workforce of clinicians, mental health professionals, allied professions, multi-disciplinary teams and diverse experts. Coherent workforce planning has secured this capacity for the long term.

Table 3.2: Interconnecting themes for the NHS Confederation and Centre for Mental Health's vision for mental health, autism and learning disability in 2032 (continued)

Theme	Description
10. Outcomes that matter	The system will no longer be driven by the outputs that matter to institutions, but by the outcomes that matter to people.

Source: Bell and Pollard (2022, pp 5–6)

- A national transitions strategy for our most vulnerable young people, ensuring they can transition into adulthood with the right care and support
- A public health-led approach to addressing drug and alcohol addictions, including access to care and treatment for those with a dual diagnosis
- By 2026, use 1% of what we spend on health to support the mental health of our young people through Child & Adolescent Mental Health Services (CAMHS). (Royal College of Psychiatrists, nd, p 1)

The Royal College of Psychiatrists in Scotland identified the need for the no wrong door policy in mental health services, noting that the COVID-19 pandemic's impact has been exacerbated by a mental healthcare system that can be confusing and disjointed and which creates delays to treatment. They argued that parity between physical and mental healthcare is a long way off, particularly for those with severe mental ill health. Their members have reported patients:

- Going through multiple channels to be referred to the right professional or service, only for delays in people being seen;
- Attending appointments with the wrong professional or service, resulting in being redirected back to the starting point
- Having to travel many miles to access the specialist care they need, or requiring admission outwith their local area. (Royal College of Psychiatrists, nd, p 6)

The report continued: 'To address these challenges, we need the next Scottish Government to work to ensure there is no wrong door to people with mental ill health accessing the right care, in the right place and at the right time' (Royal College of Psychiatrists, nd, p 7).

The Community Mental Health Framework for Adults and Older Adults (NHS England, 2019) calls for a move away from siloed, hard-to-reach services towards place-based, joined-up care and whole-person, whole-population approaches. In England, Surrey and Borders Partnership NHS Foundation Trust, the no wrong door policy is being used to transform community mental health services for adults and older adults with severe mental illness (NHS Surrey and Borders Partnership Foundation Trust, nd-a). A key aim is to ensure that people who would normally fall through the gaps between GP and specialist care, or who may be sent back and forth with rejected referrals, are seen quickly and easily. Any adult with a serious mental health problem can get help from their GP practice and advice from an MDT about wellbeing and coping with stress and anxiety. They are also connected with a wide range of VCSE sector services, such as employment and debt advice, and they have easy access to specialist mental health treatment if needed.

The new model of care is to be rolled out across every GP practice in Surrey and North East Hampshire by the end of 2023, the aim being to develop seamless, integrated and recovery-focused services across GPs, the third sector and social care. The service is being shaped by people with lived experience and their carers, through co-design. It saw more than 7,000 patients in the first two years, and patient satisfaction was high. Preliminary analysis in sample sites found that GPs had a reduction in referrals from primary to adult secondary care (Naylor et al, 2017).

Some challenges for the no wrong door policy have been identified. These include the need for comprehensive training of clinicians, the difficulty of integrating care while maintaining focus in each specialism, the need to form integrated care teams, the presence of funding streams that target specific disorders and the need for treatment guidelines to address specific dual disorders. However, with the right cooperation, policies and technology, the model can create a seamless, integrated approach to mental healthcare.

Role of the VCSE sector in service delivery

The VCSE sector is made up of a diverse range of organisations, many of which work alongside statutory bodies, including the NHS, to deliver mental health services in the community. The sector offers accessible and flexible support, and its contribution is recognised by healthcare professionals, service users and carers. Partnership working between the statutory and VCSE sector has been a government priority.

Work on mental health in the VCSE sector ranges from large national organisations lobbying government for policy and legislative change to small local organisations serving the mental health needs of the local community and self-help groups offering peer support. A recent study identified five types of VCSE organisation providing mental health crisis support: organisations that provide crisis support; those that provide general mental health services; those that provide population-focused support; those offering support to cope with particular life events; and those offering general services (Newbigging et al, 2020). The study found a wide range of support and specific expertise, although availability and accessibility varied. Inequalities were identified for rural communities, Black and minority ethnic communities, substance users and people who identify as having a personality disorder. However, the authors conclude that the breadth of the VCSE sector's contribution needs to be acknowledged and its role as an accessible alternative to inpatient care prioritised. Taking a whole-person approach to mental health crisis care should involve effective collaboration between the NHS, local authorities and the VCSE sector. The process must also include service users and carers. The VSCE's grounding in communities, whether defined in terms of specific populations or geographical areas, combined with a supportive ethos is highly valued.

Some VCSE organisations offer users benefits related to social interaction, which is particularly important for people with mild to moderate mental illness as it offers a sense of wellbeing and peer support. Services based in the community minimise the stigmatising effect of mental illness, avoiding unnecessary labelling and respecting confidentiality (Clement et al, 2015). People are often more comfortable using a VCSE organisation than they are accessing statutory services, as they can access holistic support as well as advice in relation to concerns around issues such as housing, education and employment. They value the role of VCSE organisations in advocating for mental health service users and helping them to navigate the complex statutory system by providing practical support and advice. A distinctive aspect of the contribution of the VCSE sector is the involvement of volunteers, including those with personal experience of mental illness, who can listen in a nonjudgemental way and validate personal experiences and emphasise recovery. This highlights the contribution of the sector as a partner of public services and a key pillar of the overall mental health ecosystem.

Taking an asset-based approach that considers benefits from the resources each holds, the VCSE sector can benefit from skills, knowledge and resources provided by the statutory sector, and the statutory sector can gain from capital resources, a workforce, and volunteering and peer support services. However, sustainability of the VCSE sector is a key issue (Newbigging et al, 2020).

Barriers to VCSE sector involvement

While VCSE organisations play a crucial part in supporting people's mental health, they rely on funding from statutory bodies (Bell and Allwood, 2019). The VCSE sector offers support that is distinctive and complementary to statutory services, but current commissioning processes and requirements can limit the ability of VCSE organisations to be innovative or work in a person-centred way. The financial risks that VCSE organisations face are well recognised and include:

- reduced funding from local government, creating more reliance on NHS and philanthropic funding;
- the practice of 'more for less' contracts, where statutory commissioners seek the same level of service for less funding;
- short-term or rolling contracts that leave organisations with little certainty about the future;
- framework agreements and contracts that are experienced as unfair, inefficient, overly complex and insecure;
- unpredictable and delayed decision making by commissioners;
- national policy decisions that can have unexpected effects on local decision making – for example, NHS England's Mental Health Investment Standard and the development of ICSs.

Some in VCSE organisations identified long-term funding as helpful to reduce the risk to organisations, while others thought long contracts could exclude them from being able to bid for work, work flexibly and respond to changing needs (Baxter and Fanwood, 2020). The strength of the innovative, responsive services offered in the VCSE sector is that service users' needs are responded to quickly.

Barriers also included the time it takes to establish partnerships, owing to differences in culture between the statutory and VCSE sectors. On one hand, VCSE sector staff felt that statutory services sometimes regarded them as amateurs. On the other hand, some found that running services commissioned by the statutory sector demanded challenging new skills, such as understanding statutory responsibilities in relation to General Data Protection Regulation and safeguarding legislation. There was often not enough funding to provide training to VCSE organisations, and while larger organisations had human resources and training departments that could fill this gap to some extent, smaller organisations could find it difficult to keep up with statutory requirements. The stress of working with vulnerable mental health clients also led to burnout and high staff turnover in the VCSE sector, which meant the asset-based nature of experience and knowledge was lost.

Some organisations adapted their services to access funding. For example, where local commissioners had funding available for a specific area of mental healthcare, an organisation would set up a programme specifically to access the funding. Funding was often short term and difficult to obtain. For small organisations, there could be two weeks of intensive work to submit a tender for funding only to fail to secure it. There was also a lack of transparency about the funding process and confusion around funding pathways.

Short-term funding for the VCSE sector does not allow for building expertise over time and results in a high turnover of staff. Baxter and Fancourt (2020) identify interventions to address this, including long-term funding that supports VCSE organisations' core costs, training on the commissioning process and statutory requirements, and mentor schemes and local cooperatives to support the VCSE sector in partnership work.

However, there have historically been barriers to VCSE organisations working in partnership with each other. For many years, funding bodies have been asking that organisations offering similar or compatible services form partnerships when submitting funding applications. This is something that organisations have tended to resist due to the competition for limited resources.

In terms of partnership working between the VCSE sector and statutory bodies, The King's Fund (2023) cites research that highlights three key areas where barriers and challenges have an impact:

- commissioning, service design and delivery;
- sharing data, intelligence and insight;
- funding and sustainable investment.

However, local approaches are being developed to tackle these barriers and capture and share learning. The Norfolk and Waveney Health and Care Partnership, alongside local VCSE organisations, introduced a VCSE sector assembly to improve health and care by connecting VCSE and statutory partners in the area's ICS. The NHS, county councils and VCSE sector organisations worked together to develop the assembly and link it to the local health and wellbeing board to ensure the needs of the community are met and that the voices of smaller groups are heard (Lozito et al, 2020).

WHO (2021a) guidance for community mental health voluntary action focuses on building health and social care systems that incorporate person-centred, human rights-based, recovery-oriented approaches in community mental health services. The guidance cites good practice from around the world, including the example of Link House in the UK. Link House is a residential crisis centre for women over 18 who are experiencing a mental health crisis and would otherwise be homeless. It is part of the innovative Bristol Mental Health Network, in which 18 public and VCSE sector organisations, fully funded by the NHS, are unified in the delivery of care. Link House can accommodate ten women at a time for a maximum of four weeks. The primary aim is to divert women in crisis away from emergency psychiatric hospital admission. All women experiencing a mental crisis are accepted, including those under legal treatment orders and those being discharged from psychiatric care. It uses a social care model of recovery and emphasises a strengths-based approach, valuing lived experience and self-determination. In 2017–18, Missing Link helped a total of 864 women find services and housing in their community, with 150 of them using Link House. The cost of delivering the service, including buildings, staff and overhead expenses, was £467,000 for the year. A cost comparison showed that the total cost per person per night was £127, while a hospital bed cost approximately three times more. Therefore, the service provided by Link House represented a major saving for the health system (WHO, 2021a).

The *NHS Long Term Plan* (NHS, 2019) makes a commitment to working with VCSE organisations to support people in their local community to maintain health and wellbeing. The sector has more recently been recognised as a key partner in addressing health inequalities and improving outcomes in population health, and in enhancing productivity and value for money in healthcare (NHS England and Improvement, 2021).

Individual Placement and Support

Individual Placement and Support is an evidence-based employment support intervention involving intensive individual support to help people with serious mental illness get and keep a paid job. Individuals complete a rapid job search, followed by placement in paid employment and in-work support for both the new employee and their employer. Provision of Individual Placement and Support services across England was a key commitment of the *Five Year Forward View for Mental Health* (Mental Health Taskforce, 2016). The intervention involves direct, bespoke support for employment that does not exclude people on the basis of a diagnosis. It is argued that this approach allows practitioners to engage with authentic recovery practice. The benefits have been validated by nearly three decades years of research in different countries (Metcalfe and Drake, 2021). If fully adopted and properly funded, it may be a key way of supporting mental health system reform.

ICSs

Key to integrated health and social care in England are ICSs, established following the Health and Care Act 2022. These are partnerships in which organisations come together to plan and deliver health and care services for people in the local area. Forty-two ICSs were established across England. These are responsible for allocating the NHS budget and commissioning services to meet local health needs. The legislation requires greater collaboration with system partners, and the ICSs must take account of and work with organisations that contribute to the aim of addressing the health and social care needs of the local population. The composition of ICSs is summarised in Table 3.3.

According to a study commissioned by the Association of Mental Health Providers, the VCSE sector is the largest provider of mental health services in the community, with around 1.5 million people accessing services in 2018 (Bell and Allwood, 2019). In September 2021, the NHS, acknowledging the importance of the VCSE sector, published guidance for ICSs related to implementing partnerships, noting that:

- The VCSE sector is a key strategic partner with an important contribution to make in shaping, improving and delivering services,

Table 3.3: Structure of integrated care systems

Component	Description
Integrated care partnerships	These are statutory committees jointly formed between the NHS integrated care board and all upper-tier local authorities that fall within the ICS area. They bring together a broad alliance of partners with their membership, which is determined locally. They are responsible for producing an integrated strategy on how to meet the health and wellbeing needs of the population in their ICS area.
Integrated care boards	Statutory NHS organisations are responsible for developing a plan for meeting the health and wellbeing needs of the population. They also manage the NHS budget and arrange for the provision of health services in the ICS area. Integrated care boards replaced clinical commissioning groups.

Source: NHS England (2021)

and developing and implementing plans to tackle the wider determinants of health.

- VCSE [sector] partnership should be embedded in how the ICS operates, including through involvement in governance structures in population health management and service redesign work, and in system workforce, leadership and organisational development plans. (NHS England and NHS Health Improvement, 2021, p 4)

By April 2022, integrated care boards were expected to have developed a formal agreement for engaging and embedding the sector in system-level governance and decision-making arrangements, ideally through an alliance that reflected the diversity of the sector. These arrangements were to build on the involvement of VCSE partners in relevant forums at place and neighbourhood level (NHS England and NHS Health Improvement, 2021).

The foreword to the guidance for ICSs highlighted the contribution of the VCSE sector to local communities during the COVID-19 pandemic. The most successful initiatives were those that bridged the traditional divisions between statutory health and social care and the

VCSE sector. The example of the 'Wigan Deal' showed the value of an approach where a social contract was created between citizens and state, bringing communities and local partnerships together. Part of this involved an 'invest to save' approach to strengthen the role of the VCSE sector in prevention and community resilience. A community investment fund was set up for the VCSE sector, and council officers were given the freedom to work with communities in an innovative way. The council carried out a cost-benefit analysis that estimated for every £1 the fund spent, £2 of value was created through direct savings to social care, crisis savings and benefits payments. The following lessons were highlighted:

- Find out what's important to residents and listen closely to communities. They will make the right decisions about their own lives with the right support.
- Invest in local community grassroots organisations and relationships with families to truly help people and reduce demand for expensive, ineffective and clunky state solutions.
- Give the freedom to test new approaches in integrated place-based teams. [...] Trust public servants to work with people.
- Reduce time and money spent on passing people around the system for further assessment and referrals to another agency to deal with part of their problems. (NHS England and NHS Health Improvement, 2021, pp 5–6)

A report by The King's Fund on barriers to the sector when working with ICSs argued that the scale and contribution of the sector qualifies it to play a key role in finding solutions and addressing local and system issues (Gilburt and Ross, 2023). However, to be effective, ICS leaders need to engage sector partners as system partners. A way to achieve this is to develop alliances between sectors, with groups of organisations coming together with a common set of aims or principles. This would provide ICSs with a single point of contact for communication and engagement, facilitating involvement at system and neighbourhood level in each area. Alliances between organisations are intended to allow the sectors to work in a coordinated way and maximise contribution and impact within an ICS area. NHS England has provided funding to ICSs to support and develop system-level sector alliances.

Implications include the need for commissioners to learn from the challenges experienced by VCSE organisations to assess how longer and larger contracts at ICS level might affect the sustainability and diversity of the VCSE sector, particularly smaller organisations and user-led groups within it (NHS England, 2023). The knowledge and expertise of the sector needs to be recognised in commissioning and service development processes. There is a need to work collaboratively with the sector at the earliest stage of the planning process, particularly to plan for service users who have historically been poorly served by mainstream services. Finally, there is an opportunity for statutory commissioners and VCSE providers to achieve a shared understanding of impact. Where outcome-based contracts are already in place, there may be opportunities to review and better understand how impact can be measured in a multi-sector partnership. Outcome-based accountability must be based on measured outcomes rather than aspirations. Monitoring and evaluation of service delivery outcomes is something the VCSE sector is adept at, as this is normally a requirement of both statutory and philanthropic funding bodies.

During the COVID-19 pandemic, relationships between the VCSE sector, local authorities and statutory services were tested. Collaborations within ICSs are starting to diminish the competitiveness between VCSE organisations that was necessary when they were tendering for the same funding streams. Contracting processes should not force VCSE organisations to compete for scarce short-term resources or make them afraid to say when a project needs to be adapted to accommodate unforeseen developments.

VCSEs based in the local community are trusted, accessible and can respond quickly in crisis situations. However, for the flexibility and innovation the sector can offer to be fully realised, those commissioning services from them also need to be flexible and trust the innovative social assets they possess; otherwise, the advantages to service users will be lost. For example, if a statutory commissioner is funding a mental health organisation to provide talking therapies, the organisation needs to have the autonomy to judge how many sessions an individual needs, rather than the commissioner stipulating the number of sessions.

Conclusion

Throughout the UK, healthcare is facing unprecedented demand, and this includes mental healthcare. The number of people with mental illness continues to rise, and there has been an increase in the number of children and young people accessing mental health services. Services have struggled to accommodate the numbers seeking help, and long waits to access services have become commonplace. VCSE organisations make significant contributions to mental health services. These organisations are generally viewed as being close to the communities they serve, and they are valued for their flexibility, responsiveness and creativity.

It is clear that parity of esteem for mental and physical healthcare in the UK is aspirational rather than a reality, illustrated by the fraction of spending at central government and local commissioning levels when compared to acute hospital services. A decade of underfunding even before the COVID-19 pandemic has constrained what mental health services can provide. Embedding a recovery ethos across mental health services requires a seismic shift in ideas and practices. The gap between the aspiration of recovery-based services and what is actually being delivered suggests that there is still extensive work to do to challenge prevailing assumptions, beliefs and values around mental illness.

Further reading

Carbonell, A., Navarro-Perez, J.J. and Mestre, M.V. (2020) 'Challenges and barriers in mental healthcare systems and their impact on the family: a systematic integrative review', *Health & Social Care in the Community*, 28(5): 1366–79.

House of Commons Committee of Public Accounts (2023) *Progress in Improving NHS Mental Health Services: Sixty-Fifth Report of Session 2022–23* [Online], Available at: https://publications.parliament.uk/pa/cm5803/cmselect/cmpubacc/1000/report.html (Accessed 15 July 2024).

4

The rise of the service user movement and the concept of recovery

Introduction

The antipsychiatry movement in Britain and the US in the late 1960s and 1970s led to the rise of the 'user movement' and advocacy and lobbying organisations. Some people who had been service users began calling themselves 'survivors' of mental health treatment. In the UK, there is now a political consensus that people who use public services should be involved in the design and delivery of these services, and this is in line with the key aim of the user movement to ensure greater collaboration and a move away from a paternalistic model of service provision.

More recently, the concept of 'co-production' has emerged as a value-driven approach to service delivery. It is built on the principle that those who are affected by services and have 'lived experience' are best placed to inform the planning and design of care. The nature of 'user involvement' is ambiguous and there is ongoing debate about both definition and the extent to which this idea has fundamentally changed approaches to care.

Alongside debates about how policies are shaped, the concept of 'recovery' has risen to prominence in the field of mental health. While there is no consensus on what the term means, it is generally understood to be about gaining hope and an understanding of one's abilities. It emphasises resilience and living a meaningful life. Recovery is not just about individual responses or a personal journey, but also how this relates to wider society and human rights.

Antipsychiatry

The term 'antipsychiatry' was first used by David Cooper in 1971 to describe opposition to the psychiatry of the time. The antipsychiatry movement was prevalent in Britain and the US in the 1960s and 1970s. Among its main protagonists were R.D. Laing and David Cooper in the UK, Thomas Szasz in the US, Erving Goffman in Canada and Michel Foucault in France.

As a sociologist, Goffman's (1961) analysis of asylums – which he described as 'total institutions' – was not a direct attack on psychiatry, but rather challenged social constructions of power and control. The power and control he witnessed in asylums, he argued, could also be applied to contexts such as prisons, boarding schools, ships and monasteries. Control was also identified by the French philosopher Michel Foucault (1961) in relation to the use of power and knowledge.

Laing, Cooper, and Szasz were all psychiatrists who questioned not only psychiatric treatments but also the existence of mental illness itself. Cooper (1967) argued that psychosis is due to the disparity between a person's true identity and their social identity. Laing (1960) proposed an alternative approach to patients with psychosis, who he believed struggle with confusion when experiencing contradictory messages about the world around them. He called this approach 'existential phenomenology'; it involved engaging fully with the patient rather than taking a neutral diagnostic approach.

Szasz accused psychiatrists of fabricating mental illness for their own professional advancement and labelling people as mentally ill for being social pests whose behaviour is challenging (Porter, 2002). Foucault (1961) similarly argued that mental illness must be understood as a cultural construct that had been sustained by psychiatric practices. Szasz was Professor of Psychiatry at the State University of New York Medical Centre in Syracuse when he wrote the classic *The Myth of Mental Illness: Foundations of a Theory of Personal Conduct* (Szasz, 1961). In it, he described mental illness as metaphorical illness, as illness could only affect the body and there was no such thing as illness of the mind. Therefore, there could be no treatment or cure and no medical, moral or legal justification for involuntary psychiatric intervention or hospitalisation. He believed the relationship between psychiatrist and patient should be consensual rather than coercive.

Szasz has been accused of turning against his own specialty in challenging the mental health practice of the decades after World War Two. Szasz was cited in legal cases that led to a focus on autonomy and rights for mental patients. As a result of the political influence of advocacy groups, there were sweeping changes to laws in the US that shifted decision-making powers for patient care from health professionals to lawyers. In addition, court cases led to a curtailment of the ability of doctors to commit patients to psychiatric hospitals and a move toward more autonomy for patients, who could now refuse hospitalisation. A person's need for treatment was no longer sufficient to force them into hospitalisation against their wishes. Szasz has been blamed for the deinstitutionalisation of mental health in the US, which contributed to homelessness, and he has been described as one of the most hated figures in contemporary psychology (Williams and Caplan, 2012).

Among the criticisms of the antipsychiatry academics, sociologist Kathleen Jones has cautioned that there are some serious points for psychiatry to consider in relation to their 'rhetorical excesses' and 'studied irrationality' (Turner et al, 2015, p 618). She said that the patient's view of what is happening to them is as valid as the perspective of their therapist, arguing that therapists need to listen as well as prescribe (Jones, 1978 in Turner et al, 2015). At the time, British psychiatry was 'ambivalent about Laing and generally hostile to Szasz' (Turner et al, 2015, p 618). However, when Laing died in 1989, many psychiatrists entering the profession were hoping to establish an empathetic bond with their patients, so by then Laing's contribution was regarded as welcome (Turner et al, 2015).

The rise of the user movement

The user movement in England can be traced back to the 1620s with the 'Petition of the Poor Distracted Folk of Bedlam' (Bethlem

Hospital). The Alleged Lunatics' Friend Society was set up in 1845, its aim being 'the protection of the British Subject from unjust confinement on the grounds of mental derangement and the redress of persons so confined'.

In the 1960s and early 1970s, antipsychiatry groups began to form, some of which were alliances between patients and professionals. Their emergence was influenced by Laing, Szasz and Cooper, and they gained support from a wide range of people who were becoming aware of what were perceived as abuses of power by psychiatrists. This included lobotomy, insulin coma therapy and electroconvulsive therapy, which were viewed as oppressive and thought to be used to coerce patients into behaving in certain ways. The treatment of LGBTQ+ people was also abhorrent. To 'cure' them, they were given religious counselling, psychoanalysis and aversion therapy that included inducing vomiting, and they were prescribed oestrogen to reduce libido (Bourke, 2021). A range of other user issues were raised, such as improving conditions for psychiatric patients in hospital, the closure of long-stay psychiatric hospitals and giving service users a greater say in choices relating to their quality of life (Wallcroft and Bryant, 2003). Service movements in the early 1970s were demanding civil and economic rights for patients in the community.

By the early to mid-1980s, local user forums were being formed to offer mutual support and user involvement. Groups were often small and transient, but the movement has expanded rapidly from around 12 groups in the mid-1980s to over 500 by 2005. Many of these were for carers as well as service users. Some ex-patients began to describe themselves as 'survivors' of mental health services rather than ex-users or ex-patients.

In 1985, Roy Porter, a medical historian, published his seminal article 'The patient's view: doing medical history from below', a call to give patients a voice in the writing of their own history. This was at a time when psychiatry was being challenged by new professions involved in mental health services. There was an intrusion by policy makers into mental health services, the rise of an assertive service user movement and charities advocating for mental health patients. For instance, mental health charities such as the National Schizophrenia Fellowship (now Rethink) and the National Association for Mental Health (now Mind) were in existence at the time. Groups run by patients included the Community Organisation for Psychiatric Emergencies, Protection for the Rights of Mental Patients in Treatment and the Campaign Against Psychiatric Oppression.

By the late 1990s, many mental health professionals believed that the process of deinstitutionalisation was failing due to being under-resourced, while for service users the concern was the emphasis on control and confinement, due to a few high-profile homicides carried out by patients discharged from psychiatric care. New procedures in the Mental Health Act 1983 promised more choice to service users, but it remained the case that detainees were unlikely to be successful in challenging their detention, and voluntary patients risked being detained if they did not agree with the treatment prescribed for them (Turner et al, 2015).

Despite its prominence, there is considerable debate about what user involvement means and who it refers to. As Arnstein (1969) points out in her influential ladder of citizen participation in the planning process, user involvement exists across a spectrum from informing through to co-designing, and it is closely related to ideas of power and control.

Common themes in the user movement are taking back to the power of psychiatry, rights protection and advocacy, and self-determination. While activists in the movement may to some extent share a collective identity, views exist along a continuum from conservative to radical in relation to psychiatric treatment, and there are also different levels of resistance to being viewed as a patient.

According to Millar et al (2015), there are five key attributes of service user involvement in mental healthcare:

• a person-centred approach – this includes empathy and respectful listening dignity and respect;
• informed decision-making – this relates to assessment, risk assessment, medication and treatment, and care planning;

- advocacy – this includes citizen advocacy and self-advocacy, and it addresses power imbalance;
- obtaining service user views and feedback – this addresses discrepancies between service user and practitioner views;
- working in partnership – this might be with practitioners and peer workers.

Estimates of the success of the user movement vary considerably. Pilgrim and Waldron (1998) suggest that success has been at best modest, with little impact on the development of interventions and care. Imbalances in terms of power and knowledge validation mean that service users remain marginalised in the policy-making process. Others, such as Diamond et al (2003), argue that progress has been made in acknowledging and integrating user perspectives. However, notwithstanding the advances made in recognising the value of user voices, challenges remain in terms of a tokenistic approach to legitimisation of user perspectives.

Mad studies and the mad movement

The social and academic mad movement, led by survivors, is in its early stages of development (Beresford, 2019). Mad studies originated in Canada at Ryerson and York universities in Toronto, but it is growing as a global movement. It refers to 'mental distress' rather than mental illness or disorder. It rejects the biomedical approach and is defined as 'a field of scholarship, theory, and activism about the lived experiences, history, cultures, and politics about people who may identify as Mad, mentally ill, psychiatric survivors, consumers, service users, patients, neurodiverse, and disabled' (Castrodale, 2015 in Beresford, 2019, p 1337).

However, it is not without its critics within the user/survivor movement. The most obvious objection from many of them is to do with the terminology used. Beresford et al (2010), referring to themselves as 'survivor researchers', carried out two small surveys to explore the understanding of mental health issues in society. Most who responded found the biomedical model stigmatising and connected their mental distress to social causes, such as poverty, stigma and isolation. On the idea of reclaiming the terminology, some saw this as similar to the way the LGBTQ+ community reclaimed the word 'queer', but opinion was divided, with others not wanting to embrace a term that has been associated with insult and derision.

Mad studies are described as a movement, a discipline and a form of activism. It is 'the first survivor-led movement that has sought to develop strong philosophical and theoretical principles' (Beresford and Rose, 2023, p 5). It values and prioritises lived experience and knowledge, seeks to build alliances beyond mental health, and is led by but not confined to survivors (Beresford and Rose, 2023).

The aspirations of users of mental health services are now well established, not least due to the efforts of the service user/survivor movement and the contribution in 'Mad Studies' of academics in the field. Policy makers are using the terms 'person-centred care', 'co-production' and 'user involvement' in social and mental healthcare. Service user/survivor movements, voluntary, community and social enterprise (VCSE) sector organisations and mental healthcare advocates increasingly refer to 'lived experience'. Whatever term is used, can it be assumed that the individuals in question will not need to be asking for the same basic right to have their voices heard in another decade? Can it also be hoped that those with a mental illness can access the help they need, when they need it, rather than being placed on a waiting list for treatment, with the risk that they will have died by suicide before they are seen by statutory mental health services?

Self-harm and suicide

Self-harm, defined as any act of self-poisoning or self-injury, and suicide are global health concerns. Research demonstrates that acts of self-harm are highly prevalent among adolescents and one of the strongest predictors of suicide (Moran et al, 2012; Farbstein et al, 2022). International community-based studies estimate that approximately 10–30 per cent of adolescents self-harm (Hawton et al, 2012) and 1–10 per cent report having made a suicide attempt at least once in their life (Moran et al, 2012).

Self-harm

Self-harm is an act with a non-fatal outcome in which the individual intentionally damages or injures their body as a means of expressing deep negative feelings, such as low self-esteem. Self-harm is usually an expression of personal distress rather than an illness, although it can be linked to other mental health conditions. The act of self-harm releases endorphins, providing temporary relief. This can become addictive, and over time the effects can become less effective, meaning that the pain involved needs to be more intense to provide the same effect – this increases the risk of suicidal behaviour (Cole-King and O'Neill, 2018). The UK has one of the highest rates of self-harm in Europe, and rates in England have risen since 2000, particularly among young people. Non-fatal self-harm (with or without suicidal intent) is one of the most common reasons for attendance at Accident and Emergency (A&E) and acute hospital admissions. Between 1 April 2020 and 31 March 2023 there were estimated to be over 200,000 hospital attendances for self-harm, although most incidents happen in the community and do not lead to hospital attendance (NHS Digital, February 2023).

A self-harm registry was introduced in Northern Ireland in 2012, administered by the Public Health Agency. It has played a key role in providing information for policy development and service design. According to the registry, in 2019–20, acts of self-harm and thoughts of self-harm or suicide accounted for 14,641 attendances at A&E in Northern Ireland. Almost two thirds (61 per cent) of these were due to self-harm (The Public Health Agency, 2022). Incidence rates for A&E attendance for suicide ideation increased by 5 per cent in 2019–20 compared with the previous year, and this was 79 per cent higher than in 2012–13. The rate of suicide ideation increased by 72 per cent for males and by 90 per cent for females.

Self-harm is on a continuum of suicidal behaviour, and once a person has self-harmed, their likelihood of dying by suicide increases 30 to 100 times compared to someone who has never self-harmed. Among those who attend hospital after self-harming, 1 in 50 repeat within a year, and more than 50 per cent of people who die by suicide have self-harmed. Those who self-harm have a higher mortality rate from all causes, not just suicide (Royal College of Psychiatrists, 2020).

Suicide

Suicide is usually due to complex factors rather than a single cause. It may be to do with relationship breakdown, financial worries, or health issues, either mental or physical. Globally, more than 700,000 people die by suicide every year. Furthermore, for each suicide, there are more than 20 suicide attempts (WHO, 2023). Suicide and suicide attempts have a ripple effect that impacts on families, friends, colleagues, communities and societies. However, it is important to remember that suicide is preventable and much can be done to prevent suicide at individual, community, and national levels (WHO 2023). Key to suicide prevention is compassion, hope, safeguarding, safety planning and mitigating risk factors while addressing mental illness and life crises (Cole-King, and O'Neill, 2018).

Over two thirds of people who die by suicide have not been in contact with a mental health professional or been diagnosed with a mental illness. In the UK between 2010 and 2020, only 27 per cent of all suicides were accounted for by individuals in contact with mental health services (Nuffield Trust, 2021) In their systemic review of the help-seeking behaviours of people who died by suicide, Tang et al (2021) found that being male, being in a younger or older age group, and rural location were factors associated with non-receipt of formal mental health services before death by suicide.

Suicide clusters or suicide contagion is a little-understood phenomenon that is most common in people under 25 years of age. They occur when there is a higher number of suicides than would be expected in a geographical area or in an institution, such as a school or a university. They can happen following the death of a celebrity or someone close to the individuals concerned. There is strong evidence that sensationalist reporting of suicide can lead to subsequent suicides and suicide attempts (Keyes et al, 2021).

The Samaritans (nd) provides guidance for the media when reporting suicides and self-harm:

> Research evidence shows that certain types of media depictions, such as explicitly describing a method, sensational and excessive reporting, can lead to imitational suicidal behaviour among vulnerable people. In contrast, coverage describing a person or character coming through a suicidal crisis can serve as a powerful testimony to others that it is possible and can encourage vulnerable people to seek help.

Media guidelines for the safe reporting of suicide have also been developed by the International Association for Suicide Prevention and the WHO, and this includes a list of dos and don'ts for responsible reporting by journalists:

Dos

- Do provide accurate information about where to seek help
- Do educate the public about the facts of suicide and suicide prevention, without spreading myths
- Do report stories of how to cope with life stressors or suicidal thoughts and how to get help
- Do apply particular caution when reporting celebrity suicides
- Do apply caution when interviewing bereaved family or friends
- Do recognize that media professionals themselves may be affected by stories about suicide

Don'ts

- Don't place stories about suicide prominently and don't unduly report such stories
- Don't use language that sensationalizes or normalizes suicide, or presents it as a constructive solution to problems
- Don't explicitly describe the method used
- Don't provide details about the site/location
- Don't use sensational headlines

- Don't use photographs, video footage or social media links (WHO and International Association for Suicide Prevention, 2017, p vii)

In relation to the information that can be found online, the Department of Health and Social Care invested initial seed funding of £100,000 in 2019/20 for the Samaritans to work with companies committed to establishing and funding a strategic partnership with experts in suicide and self-harm to tackle harmful content and support vulnerable users of their platforms.

Effective interventions to prevent suicide should include bereavement counselling for family and friends of a person who has died by suicide, help for susceptible individuals, engagement with media, community-based approaches to prevention and use of social media to disseminate information to young people at risk.

UK suicide profiles

Figures based on the Office for Health Improvement and Disparities Suicide Prevention profile shows that depression, a risk factor for suicide, is increasing in those aged 18.

The 2017 annual report of the National Confidential Inquiry into Suicide and Safety in Mental Health (2017), which covers mental health patients in England, Northern Ireland, Scotland and Wales, highlights new vulnerable groups. The focus in previous annual reports had been on the diagnoses found most frequently in studies of suicide – for example, depression and schizophrenia. However, the 2017 report presents figures for less common diagnoses to highlight the need for vigilance in relation to these groups. The report notes:

- Eating disorders accounted for 205 suicides in the UK between 2005 and 2015, an average of 19 deaths a year. Over two thirds had been ill for longer than five years, but only 14 were in contact with specialist eating disorder services. A history of self-harm was common, providing an important opportunity for intervention.

- Autism spectrum disorder accounted for 119 suicides in the UK between 2005 and 2015. There was an average of 11 deaths a year, though annual figures rose over the course of this period.
- Dementia accounted for 203 suicides in the UK between 2005 and 2015, and there was a steady rise from 2011. Only 32 were in the early stages of dementia (ill for less than a year).
- Carers providing care for young children or someone else at home and people living with a mental health patient accounted for 938 who died by suicide in the UK between 2005 and 2015. The average was 85 deaths a year. Carers were more likely to be female and they had fewer risk factors for suicide compared to other mental health patients.
- There were 119 suicides by people with autism spectrum disorder. Compared to all patients who died by suicide, alcohol misuse was less common for this group, and previous self-harm was more common.

The National Confidential Inquiry's annual report for 2023 provides findings relating to people aged 10 and above who died by suicide between 2010 and 2020 across all UK nations and makes recommendations for mental health clinicians to address issues identified as contributing to suicide in at-risk patients groups:

- Clinical care – patient suicide numbers and rates remained relatively stable between 2010 and 2020. It was recommended that in order to reduce numbers with sustained growing pressures, clinicians should concentrate on common factors associated with suicide, including living alone, self-harm and co-morbid alcohol and drug misuse. As loss of contact is common before suicide, it was suggested that services should actively re-establish care and involve family members where possible.
- Acute care – inpatient admission and recent discharge from hospital were periods of high risk for suicide. During 2010–20, over a quarter (28 per cent) of those who died by suicide were in acute care settings, including inpatients and people in post-discharge care and crisis resolution home treatment. Half of these patients were on agreed leave and the highest number of deaths after discharge from

psychiatric hospitals occurred on day three following discharge. It was recommended that clinical services improve patient safety at these times by removing wires or objects that could be used as a method of hanging, and ensuring that pre-discharge leave and discharge planning address any adverse circumstances the patient is returning to.

- Economic adversity – with rising costs of living in the UK, patients were likely to be at added risk for suicide. It was suggested that frontline staff should be aware of the risks involved in loss of jobs, benefits and housing, among other issues, and that they should have necessary information to signpost patients to sources of financial help and advice.
- Patients under 25 – there was an increase in suicide among young people aged 10–24 years in the general population, and this was also reflected in mental health patients. Patients under 18 and those aged 18–24 showed different characteristics and risks relevant to prevention. It was suggested that for patients under 18, the role of family and educational environments and the management of anxiety and autism are particularly important. For those aged 18–24, prevention should involve the treatment of severe mental illness and substance misuse. Self-harm services were seen as crucial for all in the under-25 age group.
- Diagnosis of personality disorder – there was an increase in patients given a diagnosis of personality disorder from 2010. These patients accounted for 11 per cent of all patient suicides between 2010 and 2020. The majority (57 per cent) were female. Women with diagnosis of personality disorder were more likely to be younger, living alone, unemployed and homeless than women with different diagnoses. Both men and women diagnosed with a personality disorder had a history of self-harm and alcohol and/or drug misuse. Historically, this group of patients have been excluded from services, and it was suggested there is a need for better models of safe and compassionate care to take account of their needs.
- Patients who identify as LGBTQ+ – LGBTQ+ patients were younger than other patients and a high proportion had experienced childhood abuse. Self-harm and a personality disorder diagnosis

were common in this group. It was suggested that clinicians should be aware of the prejudice people in this group may have experienced and other factors that may contribute to suicide risk for them. As many have a history of abuse, psychological therapies addressing trauma should be offered.

• Suicide-related internet use: in 8 per cent of all patient suicides, there was evidence of suicide-related internet use, including obtaining information on suicide methods, visiting pro-suicide websites and communicating suicide intent online. This was more likely for patients aged 25–44 (42 per cent) and 45–64 (33 per cent); this practice was found for 18 per cent of patients under 25. It was suggested that clinicians need to be aware that suicide-related internet use is a feature of suicide by patients of all ages. It can take different forms, including the promotion of suicide methods. It was suggested that enquiry about exposure to internet risks should be part of clinical assessment.

Cross-country comparison

In 2020, Scotland had the highest rate of suicide of all the UK nations (14.8 per 100,000), followed by Northern Ireland (13.3), Wales (10.3) and England (10.0). However, in 2021, Northern Ireland had the highest rate, at 14.3 per 100,000; this was only slightly higher than Scotland at 14.0, while England and Wales had the lowest rates, both at 10.5. However, it should be noted that cross-country comparisons are affected by differences in data collection and collation processes.

Suicide prevention strategies

Health and social care are a devolved matter in Northern Ireland, Scotland and Wales, and each has its own suicide and self-harm prevention strategies.

England

The National Suicide Prevention Strategy – *Preventing Suicide in England: A Cross-Government Outcomes Strategy to Save Lives* – was first published in 2012 with key aims to reduce the suicide rate in the general population and support those bereaved or affected by suicide. It identified six areas for action (Department of Health, 2012), with a seventh added in 2017 (HM Government, 2017):

1. Reduce the risk of suicide in key high-risk groups.
2. Tailor approaches to improve mental health in specific groups.
3. Reduce access to the means of suicide.
4. Provide better information and support to those bereaved or affected by suicide.
5. Support the media in delivering sensitive approaches to suicide and suicidal behaviour.
6. Support research, data collection and monitoring.
7. Reduce rates of self-harm as a key indicator of suicide risk.

The Five Year Forward View for Mental Health published in February 2016 for the NHS in England by the independent Mental Health Taskforce sets out a ten-year plan for the transformation of mental health services. It included a commitment to reduce the rate of suicide in England by 10 per cent (compared to 2015) by 2020. Although *The NHS Long Term Plan* (NHS, 2019) claimed this target would be met, the rate of suicide in England in 2020 was similar to the rate in 2015 (Balogun and Garratt, 2022).

The *Cross-Government Suicide Prevention Workplan* (HM Government, 2019) committed every government department to act on suicide and set out key deliverables and time frames monitored against commitments in the National Suicide Prevention Strategy. Funding of £57 million was allocated for suicide prevention work up to 2023/24, to support local suicide prevention plans and establish suicide bereavement and support services. From April 2019, all local authorities in England have had suicide prevention plans in place.

The fifth progress report on implementation of the national strategy (HM Government, 2021a) set out additional government funding for suicide prevention following the pressures caused by the pandemic. This included £5 million for VCSE organisations in 2021/22, to support their suicide prevention work. However, the report stated that funding alone is not enough and there needs to be a collective approach with a single agreed strategy across national and local government and the VCSE sector to drive progress in reducing suicides.

Scotland

Previous strategies in Scotland include *Choose Life: A National Strategy and Action Plan to Prevent Suicide in Scotland* (Scottish Government, 2002) and the *Suicide Prevention Strategy 2013–2016* (Scottish Government, 2013). *Every Life Matters: Scotland's Suicide Prevention Action Plan* (Scottish Government, 2018) was designed to continue the work from the 2013–16 suicide prevention strategy. It was noted in the ministerial foreword to *Every Life Matters* that Scotland had made progress in the past decade, as between 2002–06 and 2013–17 the rate of death by suicide had fallen by 20 per cent. This 'strong downward trend in suicide rates in Scotland' coincided with the earlier strategies. The target set for *Every Life Matters* was for a further reduction of 20 per cent by 2022 from a 2017 baseline. However, available data suggests there has been little change between 2018 and 2020 (National Records of Scotland, 2021).

A key action of *Every Life Matters* was the establishment of the National Suicide Prevention Leadership Group in 2018. *Every Life Matters* was extended for a year in June 2021, until a new suicide prevention strategy was published. *Creating Hope Together: Scotland's Suicide Prevention Strategy 2022–2032* was published in September 2022 (Scottish Government, 2022c). It is a ten-year strategy by the Scottish Government and COSLA (the Convention of Scottish Local Authorities). This strategy aims to ensure that efforts to tackle issues such as poverty, debt and addiction include measures to address suicide.

Wales

A five-year national action plan, *Talk to Me*, was published in 2009 by the Welsh Government. A review of progress by Public Health Wales in 2012 found that the inclusion of a large number of supporting actions had reduced focus on delivery of actions specific to suicide and self-harm. The National Advisory Group to the Welsh Government on suicide and self-harm prevention were asked to redraft the plan, and the strategy and action plan *Talk to Me 2: Suicide and Self Harm Prevention Strategy for Wales 2015–2020* was launched in July 2015. (Welsh Government, 2015)

A midpoint review of *Talk to Me 2* was conducted in March 2018 (Public Health Wales, 2018) to measure progress, and this concluded that excellent progress had been made in developing local suicide prevention action plans. Good progress had been made in improving awareness, knowledge and understanding of suicide and self-harm, supporting the media in sensitive reporting of suicide and reducing access to the means of suicide. Some progress had been made in delivering appropriate responses to personal crises, early intervention and management, information and support for those bereaved or affected by suicide and self-harm, and support for learning, information and monitoring systems and research to improve understanding and guide actions. The review concluded that very little funding had been available to support the implementation, coinciding with a period of financial constraint within the health service, but there had been progress and guidance and outcomes were delivered.

Northern Ireland

Northern Ireland's first suicide prevention strategy and action plan, covering 2006–11, *Protect Life: A Shared Vision*, was published in October 2006 (Department of Health, Social Services and Public Safety, 2006) with a refreshed version published in June 2012 to cover the period 2011–13 (Department of Health, Social Services and Public Safety, 2012b). An evaluation of the implementation of the 2006 strategy (Department of Health, Social Services and Public Safety, 2010) found it had been successful in two of its aims:

- raising awareness of mental health issues with a public information media campaign and media guidelines to ensure suicide was reported sensitively;

- enhancing the support role of the VCSE sector in supporting bereaved families and people who had made previous suicide attempts.

Early recognition and intervention with follow-up support services was not wholly achieved due to variable awareness of support services among primary care providers.

The first *Protect Life* strategy in 2006 had identified depression, drug misuse, personality disorder, hopelessness, low self-esteem, bereavement, relationship breakdown and social isolation as suicide risk factors. However, in 2016 it was found that the most common risk factors were economic problems and recent self-harm.

Following an eight-week public consultation, *Protect Life 2* was launched in September 2016 in draft form (as there was no health minister in place at the time due to the Northern Ireland Assembly being in suspension). During the consultation, the Department of Health had considered whether the 'purpose' of the strategy should include self-harm, which had not been included in the 2016 purpose statements to 'reduce suicide in the north of Ireland' and 'reduce the differential in the suicide rate between the most deprived areas and the least deprived areas'. This decision was criticised, as self-harm and A&E attendance are known to be precursors to suicide (O'Neill et al, 2019).

Protect Life 2: A Strategy for Preventing Suicide and Self Harm in Northern Ireland 2019-2024 was finally published in September 2019 (Department of Health (Northern Ireland), 2019). This is a cross-departmental long-term strategy for reducing suicide and self-harm. It stresses the importance of services, communities, families and society in helping to prevent suicide. In practice, this will mean:

> that community and voluntary organisations are supported to deliver suicide prevention services; that sports clubs and faith groups are trained in suicide awareness and intervention; that justice services develop and implement self-harm and suicide prevention action plans; that primary health care is skilled and proactive in identifying and intervening with patients showing signs of suicidal behaviour; that there is closer working with

addiction services; that schools know how to respond when a pupil is in emotional distress; and that those delivering public services to potentially vulnerable people are trained in suicide awareness. (Department of Health (Northern Ireland), 2019, p 6)

A progress report in March 2023 cautioned that the full implementation of all *Protect Life 2* strategy actions was dependent on further investment (Department of Health (Northern Ireland), 2023).

VCSE sector role in suicide prevention

Suicide prevention in the UK includes initiatives by the VCSE sector. A study carried out in Northern Ireland (Jordan et al, 2011) to understand suicidal behaviour in young men aged 16–34 found that the type, nature and geographical location of formal mental health services offered only limited help for young men with suicidal thoughts and behaviours. The types of environment where they felt most comfortable were non-statutory, community-based services. It was recommended that proactive services should be based in the community, located in non-mental health environments like sports clubs, workplaces, schools and community interest and self-help groups, and there should be open access. Findings confirmed that community-based informal drop-in centres were more in line with how young men wanted to interact socially. Peer groups were seen as important so that people could be exposed to people who were no longer suicidal and could discuss the impact of suicide on friends and family and show that recovery is possible (Betts and Thompson, 2017).

Person-centred care and co-production

The National Health Service and Community Care Act 1990 was the first piece of UK legislation to make user involvement a requirement in service planning, and this marked an important change in government thinking on the role of service users. The *National*

Service Framework for Mental Health in 1999 and *The NHS Plan* in 2000 (NHS Health Education) further emphasised the role of service users as key stakeholders in service provision.

In 2009, a report stated that co-production was a new way of thinking about public services and had the potential to deliver a major shift in how health, education, policing and other services are delivered, making them much more effective and efficient, and therefore more sustainable (Boyle and Harris, 2009). At the time, co-production was predicted to become the most important revolution in public services since the Beveridge Report in 1942. However the report found there were four barriers stopping co-production becoming the default model for public services. The barriers identified were commissioning co-production activity, generating evidence of value, taking successful co-production approaches to scale and developing professionals' skills (Boyle and Harris, 2009).

Over a decade later, a universal definition of co-production is still being debated. The Health Innovation Network in South London provides the following definition:

> Person-centred care is about seeing the person as an individual and considering their desires, values, family and social circumstances and lifestyle and working together with professionals to develop appropriate solutions. Partnership working can happen at individual level, or in a collective group where public or patient groups are involved in decisions about the design and delivery of services. (Health Innovation Network, 2016)

NHS England's *Person-Centred Care Framework* (NHS Health Education England, 2017) aims to embed best practice and sets out core transferable behaviours, knowledge and skills. Person-centred approaches underpin existing dementia, learning disabilities, mental health and end-of-life care. These approaches can be used across services and sectors, including health, social care, local authorities and housing, and in different types of organisation across the public, private and VCSE sectors.

To change the way that health and care relate to people and communities, NHS England set out six principles, requiring that:

- care and support is person-centred: personalised, coordinated, and empowering
- services are created in partnership with citizens and communities
- focus is on equality and narrowing inequalities
- carers are identified, supported and involved
- voluntary, community and social enterprise and housing sectors are involved as key partners and enablers
- volunteering and social action are recognised as key enablers.

(NHS England, nd-b)

A scoping review to explore co-production and co-design terminology in the context of health and social care (Masterson et al, 2022) found increasing numbers of definitions in the last decade; just over a third of articles included in the review provided no definition or explanation of the concepts. There was also an increase in the number of publications using the terms co-production and co-design when there was no recorded involvement of citizens, patients or service users. The authors note that co-production and co-design are conceptualised in a wide range of ways and that, rather than seeking a universal definition of these terms, future applied research should focus on articulating the underlying principles and values that need to be translated and explored in practice. They conclude that co-production and co-design are evolving concepts with a level of uncertainty as to their definition, and they recommend listening to service users:

because if concepts that set out to share power are (inadvertently) misused, not only may assets and resources be wasted through the implementation of ineffective or inefficient service solutions but mistrust in health and social care services and/or dilution of the impact of genuine co-production and co-design approaches may result. (Masterson et al, 2022, p 910)

In an evaluation by the Social Care Institute for Excellence (SCIE) covering the first two years of a programme of co-production in adult social care in Oxfordshire County Council, the Deputy Director of Adult Social Care and Co-Chair of Oxfordshire's Team-Up Co-Production Board defined co-production as 'informing, consulting, involving and empowering to achieve equal partnership and collaboration between people who use services, carers, professionals and organisations to find shared solutions' (SCIE, 2020, p 2). The evaluation says co-production cannot be a 'bolt-on innovation', as it fundamentally changes the way public services are delivered. Its objective is to reduce need, rebuild the social infrastructure and shift the balance of power. A quote from a service user involved in the programme shows what co-production means to them:

> Co-production means to me that service users play a part in running services together with the people who provide services. It's not just an idea either, it actually is an important process where services are not just presented to people so they can take it or leave it. They play a part in constructing it. (SCIE, 2020, p 6)

The evaluation notes that co-production will only work if people at all levels of an organisation are signed up to it. This includes senior and middle management along with people working on the ground. As it is ultimately about sharing power, it requires a culture change at all levels of an organisation. As one worker in the VCSE sector said: 'There is some scepticism about how much the council will share power, because they still hold the purse strings, and make the final decision, but having everything co-produced up to that point is pretty impressive, and further than it has gone before' (SCIE, 2020, p 21).

The SCIE recommend the development of a more universal understanding of co-production. As co-production is not widely understood and often confused with 'involvement', it cannot be assumed when working on a project or with another organisation that there is a common understanding of the co-production approach (SCIE, 2020).

A study of co-production in Scotland found that although health and social care policy in Scotland extols the benefits of co-production, calling for approaches to be 'embedded, enabled and have meaning locally', there is no clarity on how to implement and deliver effective co-production (Connolly et al, 2022, p 2). Their analysis shows that although co-production is present in health and social care policy in Scotland, guidance and support is absent on undertaking co-production, including when it is appropriate, in which contexts and with whom. Despite the prominence of the concept of co-production, there is clearly little consensus about what it is, what it can achieve and the risks associated with it.

A guide to co-production was produced by the Department of Health (Northern Ireland) (2018), outlining key steps for its adoption and implementation across the health and social care system. The guide initially sets parameters in relation to patient and public safety, stating that there is a range of circumstances where co-production in decision making may not be appropriate, due to safeguarding issues for people and families who are physically, psychologically and socially vulnerable. The guide includes a table of what co-production is and what it is not (see Table 4.1).

Co-production is seen as an integral part of 'patient-centred care' and is a central tenet of policy in health and social care. However, there is no clear understanding of what it means across management and user levels, or in the different sectors expected to implement it.

According to the National Institute for Health and Care Excellence (NICE, 2016), the Care Act 2014 states that people should be in control of their care. An overarching principle is that care and support should be person-centred and focused on recovery (NICE, 2016).

Concept of recovery

The concept of recovery from mental illness emerged with deinstitutionalisation in the 1960s and 1970s and the start of the service user/survivor movement. Prior to that, mental illness had been shaped by the medical model, which focuses on controlling

Table 4.1: What co-production is and is not

Co-production is	Co-production is not
Partners respecting each other and valuing each other's perspective and contribution	Just giving people a chance to speak but not using the information
Working together from the very start to identify and achieve an end result that is collaboratively agreed on	Confrontation and 'winning and losing'
Listening to each other and understanding where everyone is coming from and the particular challenges they face	A quick fix
At times deferring to the other on grounds of practicality, economics, ethics, equality of civic rights, requirements under Section 75 (Northern Ireland's equality legislation)	Consultation – i.e. having a plan and then going out to tell people about it OR even having a plan, asking people's thoughts about it and incorporating these thoughts into a revised plan
Valuing, learning from and building on the different skills, assets, experience and expertise that different people bring to the process	One partner simply trying to persuade another to come round to their way of thinking
Working in ways that best meet the needs of all partners	Listing problems and expecting someone else to solve them
Sharing ownership for developing solutions that are evidence based, work and are deliverable	A new way to get your personal agenda on the table at the expense of someone else's
Breaking down barriers between professionals/providers and people using public services	A new forum for public service staff to tell people what is going to happen, or for people to lobby the public sector
Committing jointly to support and develop the capacity and understanding of all people involved in the process	
Trust, support and information sharing	

Table 4.1: What co-production is and is not (continued)

Co-production is	Co-production is not
Taking shared ownership when solutions don't work first time and taking a joint problem solving approach to move forward	
Talking with and not to	

Source: Department of Health (Northern Ireland) (2018, p 19)

symptoms. Recovery involves much more than recovery from illness itself. People with mental illness may have to recover from the stigma they have incorporated into their very being from the effects of treatment settings, the lack of recent opportunities for self-determination and the negative side effects of unemployment and crushed dreams. Recovery is often a complex, time-consuming process (Anthony, 1993).

In the 1980s, community support and rehabilitation programmes laid the foundation for a vision for the 1990s that promoted the concept of recovery from mental illness. In 1993, William Anthony, PhD, founder of the Centre for Psychiatric Rehabilitation at Boston University, predicted that recovery from mental illness would be the vision guiding mental health services in the 1990s, with implications for how mental health services would be designed.

Although recovery as a concept was common in physical illness, it had not received attention or been researched in the area of severe and persistent mental illness. In physical illness or disability, recovery did not necessarily mean that all symptoms were removed and the person's functioning was completely restored, and in the same way it was recognised that someone with a mental illness could recover even though the illness was not cured. Recovery involves:

a deeply personal, unique process of changing one's attitudes, values, feelings, goals, skills and/or roles. It is a way of living a satisfying, hopeful, and contributing life even with limitations caused by the illness. Recovery involves the development of new meaning and purpose in one's life as one grows beyond the catastrophic effects of mental illness. (Anthony, 1993, p 15)

Research in 2003 on the service user movement found that service users were not simply concerned with psychiatric care, but with the impact of their mental health problems on all aspects of their lives. This included tackling the stigma of mental illness, access to benefits and employment, and opportunities for social inclusion and recovery (Wallcroft and Bryant, 2003).

According to the 'recovery movement', which had sprung from the service user movement in the US in the 1970s and 1980s, people with severe mental illness understand that they are not defined by their illness. However, Cohen and Cohen (1984) refer to the opposite perspective, 'the clinicians' illusion'. Here, clinicians, as a result of frequently seeing people at the most acute stages of their mental distress, view recovery through the medical lens as the absence of the clinical symptoms. Such pessimistic professional narratives in relation to people with mental illness are in sharp contrast to a holistic understanding of recovery, with a focus on strengths, possibility and hope (Ellison et al, 2018). This divergence creates a barrier to the concept of recovery being universally accepted as the cornerstone of mental health policy and practice.

In response to an article on recovery in the May 2008 issue of *Mental Health Today*, an anonymous letter to the editor in the July/August 2008 edition was headed 'Recovery? In the voluntary sector we've been doing it for years' (Anon, 2008, p 37) . The author notes that in the late 1990s the voluntary sector was involved in establishing a service for people with mental health conditions based on the principles of a 'psycho-social/strengths/recovery model'. They argue that the sector has been promoting 'client-centred models' and that the earlier article demonstrated how little attention had been paid by mainstream mental health professionals to developments and initiatives in the sector.

In 2012, the WHO launched the QualityRights initiative, a global programme for community-based mental health services that promote person-centred, recovery-oriented and rights-based services. In many developed countries, including the UK and the US, recovery-oriented practice is central to mental health policy. Mental health policy in England has supported a focus on recovery since the beginning of the 21st century. However, recovery means different things to different people. Clinical recovery is a psychiatric term and refers to an alleviation of symptoms allowing for what would be considered 'normal' social functioning. Personal recovery is different. Personal recovery can happen without clinical recovery. The WHO defines a recovery-focused approach as 'gaining and retaining hope, understanding of one's abilities and disabilities, engagement in an active life … and a positive sense of self' (WHO, 2012, p 41).

The REFOCUS Programme (2009–14) in England aimed to make community- based adult mental health services more recovery focused. It was a programme of research that identified five core processes of recovery: connectedness, hope, identity, meaning and empowerment (the acronym being CHIME). A study to investigate the association between access to social capital and the recovery process of people with severe mental illness supported the idea that recovery could be measured and defined by service users. The findings supported previous findings that social relationships were important for mental health and wellbeing.

Roberts and Boardman (2013) describe the recovery ethos as being based on values, ideas and principles that arise in a personal, activist and political context rather than in clinical settings. It is linked to a search by people with mental illness for humane care, social justice, individual rights, citizenship, equality and freedom from prejudice and discrimination as a basis for living well. Lobbying led to mental health policy adopting recovery as one of its six overall aims, with a commitment by the Department of Health in 2011 to 'test the key features of organisational practice to support the recovery of those using mental health services' (Roberts and Boardman, 2013, p 401). This led to the Centre for Mental Health and NHS Confederation's Implementing Recovery through Organisational Change (ImROC) programme.

ImROC

ImROC was a three-year project involving the NHS, the independent sector and users/carers across 29 sites in England. The project ran during 2009–12 and delivered more than 50 joint training sessions that were 'co-produced' by service users and staff and delivered to over 400 staff, service users and managers. The programme recruited, trained and supported over 150 peer support workers, who worked alongside staff as peer trainers. The ImROC programme made the following conclusions about organisational change to implement recovery:

- methods need to be flexible enough to set locally relevant goals and managers must ensure that local users and carers are engaged as true partners, creating a culture of 'co-production';
- leadership is critical and must be delivered at different levels with existing staff being part of the solution;
- change needs effective project management at operational level that is supported by strategy at organisational level; and
- a different approach to risk assessment and management is needed to move toward a recovery-oriented approach. (Betts and Thompson, 2017, p 29)

ImROC led to the establishment of 'recovery colleges', which deliver educational courses on mental health and recovery with co-production at their core (see the next section).

In 2011, *No Health without Mental Health* was published (HM Government and Department of Health, 2011). One of its six key mental health objectives was a move towards more recovery-oriented policies and allowing people to plan their own recovery. Recovery is now a cornerstone of mental healthcare policy in the UK.

Recovery colleges

'Rarely has an idea in the mental health arena been taken up so widely or so quickly as that of a "Recovery College"' (Perkins et al, 2018, p 1). Recovery colleges implement person-centred care through co-production. The idea of recovery colleges was first raised around 2007–08, and a pilot recovery college was established in London in 2009. By 2017, there were more than 75 recovery colleges throughout the UK and internationally, in Australia, Canada, Hong Kong, Japan, the Republic of Ireland, Scandinavia and other countries in Western Europe. An international community of practice was established, and in 2017 the European Development Fund invested €7.6 million to build on existing initiatives and create a Cross-Border Recovery College Network, which serves 8,000 people facing mental health challenges in Northern Ireland and the border counties of the Republic of Ireland.

Recovery colleges offer an example of best practice in co-production. People are supported through education. The courses on offer are based on co-design, drawing on professional expertise and the lived experience of service users. Therefore, different colleges are likely to offer different courses, as they are based on the co-produced priorities of the professionals and those with lived experience who design the curriculum at the particular college. Courses might cover understanding of different mental health issues and treatments or they might explore what recovery means to the individual and how family and friends can support them. Courses often focus on strengthening competencies for self-care and the development of life skills and confidence to rebuild lives. It has been shown that recovery colleges can play an important role in reducing reliance on mental health services, as students develop the ability to manage their own mental health. It has also been found that guided self-help for depression and anxiety has effects comparable to face-to-face treatments (WHO, 2022c).

Studies emphasise several key features of recovery colleges, including co-production, co-facilitation and co-learning. These change power relationships through a progressive recovery focus, an educational approach and the opportunity for peer support. Recovery colleges also have an important role in transforming attitudes and systems across the mental healthcare system. Perkins et al (2012) outline the different approaches of education and therapy (see Table 4.2).

Table 4.2: Different approaches in therapy and education

A therapeutic approach	An educational approach
Focuses on problems, deficits and dysfunctions	Helps people recognise and make use of their talents and resources
Strays beyond formal therapy sessions and becomes the overarching paradigm	Assists people in exploring their possibilities and developing their skills
Transforms all activities into therapies – work therapy, gardening therapy, etc.	Supports people to achieve their goals and ambitions
Problems are defined, and the type of therapy is chosen, by the professional 'expert'	Staff become coaches who help people find their own solutions
Maintains the power imbalances and reinforces the belief that all expertise lies with the professionals	Students choose their own courses, work out ways of making sense of (and finding meaning in) what has happened and become experts in managing their own lives

Source: Perkins et al (2012, p 3)

Perkins et al (2012) also set out eight defining features of recovery colleges:

1. **Co-production between people with personal and professional experience of mental health problems**
   There should be co-production at every level and every stage, from initial planning and development, to decisions about operation, curriculum and quality assurance […].
2. **There is a physical base (building) with classrooms and a library where people can do their own research** […].
3. **It operates on college principles** […].
4. **It is for everyone**
   People with mental health problems, families, carers, staff from mental health service providers and people from partner agencies can all attend courses […].

5. **There is a Personal Tutor (or equivalent) who offers information, advice and guidance** […].
6. **The College is not a substitute for traditional assessment and treatment**
   A Recovery College complements specialist, technical assessment and treatment by helping people to understand their problems and learn how to manage these better in order to pursue their aspirations. It is a place where 'lived experience' is blended with the expertise of mental health practitioners […].
7. **It is not suitable for mainstream colleges**
   If it is to promote participation and citizenship the College should not substitute for the general education and opportunities offered by local educational establishments. It can, however, provide a route on to mainstream education via, for example, 'return to study' courses […].
8. **It must reflect recovery principles in all aspects of its culture and operation**
   […] The messages should be of hope, empowerment, possibility and aspirations. (Perkins et al, 2012, pp 3–5, original emphasis)

Perkins et al (2012) point out that recovery colleges have had their critics, most notably Recovery in the Bin, a user-led group for mental health survivors and supporters. They described themselves as a critical theorist and activist collective and want 'a robust "Social Model of Madness, Distress and Confusion" placing mental health within the context of social justice and the wider class struggle' (Recovery in the Bin, nd). They were fed up with co-opted 'recovery' being used to discipline and control those who are trying to find a place in the world and live as they wish as they deal daily with very real mental distress. In relation to recovery colleges, they described them as prescriptive and demanding compliance, and they said that they offer a curriculum that is not evidence-based but is a cost-cutting alternative to more effective evidence-based treatments. They also claimed recovery colleges do not genuinely reflect equality between practitioners and service users. This argument is based on the different rates of pay for peer trainers and mental health practitioner trainers. They claimed recovery colleges become segregated mental health ghettos as an alternative to mainstream colleges, and they infantilise those who use them. From this perspective, recovery colleges represent a manifestation of individualised neoliberalism and ignore the social, economic and political context of people's lives.

While research has tended to examine the impact on the mental health of students in recovery colleges, a systematic review of qualitative literature sought to ascertain whether genuine partnership working was happening in the colleges (Bester et al, 2022). For the purposes of the review, Bester et al define co-production as 'a collaborative process wherein people with lived experience of mental distress and mental health practitioners work safely together, in a position of parity throughout, to achieve a common goal' (2022, p 53).

Emerging themes important to co-production in the recovery college setting were power dynamics, practitioner attitudes and relationships with host organisations (Bester et al, 2022). Most of the recovery colleges worked with provider partnerships or host organisations. In the UK, these are usually health trusts, but they can also be colleges, universities, healthcare providers and VCSE organisations. In relation to power dynamics and practitioner attitudes, Bester et al (2022) suggest that the studies included in their review show that co-production is functioning well within recovery colleges. It has been noted that there are challenges for host organisations in implementing co-production, with the potential for the host organisation to not fully buy into the concept of co-production. However, having a recovery college closely associated with a host organisation allows the recovery college ethos to influence the host organisation in co-production working (Bester et al, 2022).

A national survey identified 88 recovery colleges operating in England in 2021 (Hayes et al, 2023). According to Hayes et al, previous reviews had suggested that recovery colleges benefit not only students but also staff and wider society, and that they are associated with attainment of recovery goals, improved quality of life and wellbeing, increased knowledge and self-management skills, reduced service use and changes in service providers' practice. However, there was little information on costs or organisational characteristics of recovery colleges.

As part of the survey by Hayes et al (2023), the RECOLLECT Fidelity Measure was designed to determine organisational and student characteristics, fidelity (a measure used to rate how well an intervention fits to a model) and funding. Questions were tailored to the student and relate to equality, adult learning, co-production, social connectedness, community focus and commitment to recovery. High fidelity scores were found, with NHS and strengths-focused colleges associated with highest fidelity. In 2021, the median annual budget was £200,000 and the median cost per student was £518. Cost per course designed was £5,566 and per course run was £1,510. The total annual budget across England for recovery colleges was an estimated £17.6 million, including £13.4 million from NHS budgets, with 11,000 courses delivered to 45,500 students. Staffing and co-production of new courses are key drivers of spending in recovery colleges. However, the estimated budget of recovery colleges was less than 1 per cent of NHS mental health spending.

Conclusion

The involvement of service users and survivors in the design, development, delivery and evaluation of mental health services is well-established. The user movement in mental health has evolved over the past five decades and mental health service users are increasingly active in influencing policy and practice. A key aim of this movement is to make services more responsive to the needs of the people who use them. However, there is ongoing debate about the extent to which user involvement actually makes a difference to services. Involvement may amount to little more than consultation, or in some cases it may deliver genuine power and control to service users.

The term co-production has become prominent in policy making. This collaborative model includes stakeholders in the design and delivery of services. Despite the wealth of reasons to co-produce, there is little consensus about what to do and how to do it.

Recovery is a contested concept. For professionals, it may mean successful treatment. For individuals with a mental illness, it may be about retaining hope and an ability to manage and understand one's own symptoms. This is a personal journey that allows the individual to know their strengths and live meaningful lives. The development of recovery colleges has been widely viewed as an important intervention that may change attitudes associated with professional practice. Courses offer an understanding of mental health issues and the opportunity to develop life skills through capacity building. However, these have provoked controversy, with some claiming that they reinforce power imbalances and ignore broader societal inequalities.

Further reading

Chassot, C.S. and Mendes, F. (2015) 'The experience of mental distress and recovery among people involved with the service user/survivor movement', *Health*, 19(4): 372–88.

Lyon, S. (2023) 'The recovery model in mental health care: person-centred, holistic approach', *Verywell Mind* [Online], 4 April, Available at: https://www.verywellmind.com/what-is-the-recovery-model-2509979 (Accessed 29 June 2024).

5

Social determinants
of mental health

Introduction

Historically, mental health issues were largely understood to be biological with genetic underpinnings, rather than related to broader social risk factors. The field of psychiatry focused on individual-level explanations, not the wider social, political and environmental risk factors. However, the importance of both social and biological factors in shaping poor mental health is increasingly accepted. Health outcomes are influenced by income, education level, relationships with friends and family, housing and politics as well as genetics. The social determinants of mental health are the social factors that disrupt optimal mental health and increase the risk and prevalence of mental illness, with worsening outcomes for individuals with mental illness. Broadly, the social determinants of mental health include economic and social policies, economic and political systems, development agendas and social norms that can positively and negatively influence the health and wellbeing of individuals and communities (WHO, 2022c). Often these issues are underpinned by an unequal and unjust distribution of opportunity, which, in turn, is driven by both public policies and social norms (Shim and Compton, 2020). It is important to understand that good mental health is a core indicator of human development, and it is necessary to integrate a mental health and psychosocial perspective into development and humanitarian policies, programmes and services, particularly those with internationally agreed goals and commitments (United Nations, 2010; WHO, 2022c).

The need to recognise the social determinants of mental health

The concept of social determinants of mental health is of central importance when assessing population health and healthcare. The WHO defines the social determinants of health as follows:

> Social determinants of health are the conditions in which people are born, grow up, live, work and age. These conditions influence a person's opportunity to be healthy, his/her risk of illness and life expectancy. Social inequities in health – the unfair and avoidable differences in health status across groups in society – are those that result from the uneven distribution of social determinants. (WHO, 2024, p 1)

Psychological distress is highly sensitive to social inequalities, and therefore it is inappropriate to treat it as a medical condition that can be cured. It has been argued that the key reason for the failure of governments to address the growing problem of mental illness is the wholesale adoption of a biomedical theory of mental 'health', which defines many forms of disease according to abnormalities in individual psychology, neurophysiology or behaviour. This biomedical stance is operationalised in policy as delivery of remedial services to treat mental illness, and it persists despite abundant evidence that mental health is significantly shaped by social conditions over the life course – in other words, the social determinants of mental health. This biomedicalism has served as a convenient mechanism to depoliticise 'health' by equating it with healthcare, separating it from broader questions about social and economic inequalities (Fisher, 2022). Additionally, this tendency to prioritise biological determinants over social determinants has an important public impact. On the one hand, it is positive in that it may reduce the attribution of blame for the disorder to the individual experiencing it. However, any positive implications of this focus are completely overshadowed by the negative consequences of the belief the person is to blame. An extensive body of evidence indicates that endorsing biological determinants over social factors is associated with lower optimism about recovery prospects and increased stigmatising attitudes. Attributing mental illness to biological factors is associated with stronger beliefs about dangerousness and a greater desire to be separate from people with mental illness (Huggard et al, 2023). Importantly, these attitudes are associated with both the general public and mental health professionals. This has important implications for the type and quality of support (Lebowitz and Applebaum, 2019).

Overemphasising biological determinants minimises the complex interplay of factors responsible for mental health problems, which can lead to poorer outcomes. Depression is a leading cause of disability worldwide and a major risk factor for suicide. It is also an illness that is extremely sensitive to the social determinants of health – worsening depressive symptoms have been associated with unemployment, adverse childhood experiences, racism, discrimination, food insecurity and various other environmental factors. Similarly, schizophrenia is associated with 'social drift', through which people with schizophrenia often end up with low levels of educational attainment, unemployed, homeless and sometimes frequently interacting with the criminal justice system. Depending on your perspective, social drift could be considered a biopsychosocial phenomenon associated with schizophrenia. A recognised consequence of this mental illness is that it makes it extremely difficult to sustain employment, housing and social relationships. However, given that prevailing social norms frequently view people with schizophrenia as unpredictable, dangerous outsiders, it is easy to see how these prejudices create circumstances in which social drift is inevitable (Shim and Compton, 2020).

Although public health stresses the significance of social determinants of health on chronic physical conditions, such as heart disease, stroke and hypertension, until quite recently there was little acknowledgment of their far-reaching impacts on mental health. While there is a vast literature on the determinants of physical health, a comparable focus in the field of mental health is relatively underdeveloped. There are several explanations for this gap. First, mental health is notoriously difficult to define and conceptualise. Definitions may depend on cultural norms and may change according to life stage or age. Second, mental health is difficult to measure or quantify. It is difficult to identify causal relationships, and this has hampered policy development. The lack of precise measures may cause scepticism about the prevalence of disorders or an overestimation of their prevalence (Summergard, 2016). The impact of stigma means individuals, to avoid being labelled, may be reluctant to admit to having mental illness. This can lead to denial, minimisation of symptoms and under-reporting of mental disorders. Third, there is a lack of robust data, particularly related to the impact of socio-economic context. Fourth, there has been a relative lack of interest in this issue at a government and policy level (Mohomed, 2020). The underprioritising of mental illness has led to an unwillingness to invest in publicly funded mental healthcare that offers person-centred, high-quality intervention and treatment. Despite repeated commitments at global level to ensure parity between physical and mental health, mental healthcare remains chronically underfunded, with substantial treatment gaps (Asher and De Silva, 2017).

The relationship between social factors and mental health is a complex interplay of a wide range of stresses and vulnerabilities. Understanding the impact of these social determinants is crucial for a number of reasons. First, it is important to understand how individual factors interact with societal factors in determining the mental health of an individual. Second, understanding the impact of social factors enables the development of effective population-level interventions to address health inequalities. Third, information about which population-level interventions are effective allows mental health initiatives to be linked to agreed targets to meet United Nations Sustainable Development Goals.

Social determinants of health and health inequities are amenable to change through policy and governance interventions. In 2005, the WHO established the Commission on Social Determinants of Health to collect evidence, inform debate and formulate policies, with the goal of improving the health of vulnerable people. The Commission argued that the gross inequalities in the health sector should be of concern to all policy makers, not just those interested in health. It aimed to develop a global movement to promote equality, recognising that huge differences in health outcomes are not inevitable and the distribution of health risks worldwide is unacceptable. The reduction of health inequalities is an ethical imperative. The Commission published its final report in August 2008, setting out three principles for action:

- 'Improve the conditions of daily life – the circumstances in which people are born, grow, live, work, and age' – governments should place an emphasis on early years and early intervention. Education and skills should be valued and resourced as they directly influence health and high-quality education equips individuals for success. Social protection policies should support all citizens. Governments should ensure that the conditions exist for a flourishing, fulfilling older life.
- 'Tackle the inequitable distribution of power, money, and resources' – this should be done internationally, nationally and globally. Poverty is often intergenerational and a result of systems that deny opportunities to some individuals.
- 'Measure the problem, evaluate action, expand the knowledge base, develop a workforce that is trained in the social determinants of health, and raise public awareness about the social determinants of health' – acting effectively on health inequalities means ensuring that there is a workforce of practitioners and policy makers trained to address the issues. (WHO, 2008, p 2)

Addressing the social determinants of mental health

The landmark *Fair Society, Healthy Lives: The Marmot Review*, published in February 2010, set out the scale of health inequalities in England and the interventions needed to address them (Marmot, 2010). A growing body of research identifies the social factors at the root of inequalities in health. Marmot argued that systemic differences in health for different groups are avoidable with reasonable interventions and that the continued existence of health inequalities is unfair and unjust. Social determinant frameworks focus on understanding how the circumstances in which people live and work shape their health outcomes. These determinants (circumstances) underpin deep-seated global health inequalities, such as lower life expectancy, higher rates of child mortality and a greater burden of disease on deprived populations.

Social determinant frameworks build on the concept of the 'social gradient', according to which people with lower social status have increased health risks and lower life expectancy than those with higher status, with the impact of social position potentially accumulating over time (Marmot and Bell, 2016). Basically, the lower the socioeconomic position, the worse the health outcomes. The poorest people have the highest levels of illness and premature death. Differences in social determinants are thought to develop from unequal distribution of resources, and this is not inevitable, but rather the result of politics and poor policies.

In their influential review of the social determinants of mental health, Allen et al (2014) applied a multilevel framework to organise evidence:

- the life-course approach across various life stages, including pre- and perinatal periods, early childhood, later childhood, working and family-building years and older age;
- community-level contexts, including the natural and built environment, primary healthcare and humanitarian settings;
- country-level contexts, including political, social, economic and environmental factors, cultural and social norms operating within a specific society and whether specific policies and strategies exist to reduce social inequalities and promote access to education, employment, healthcare, housing and other services.

Allen et al (2014) conclude that deprived and marginalised populations are most affected by mental disorders, with cumulative stress and physical health serving as mechanisms through which the impacts of these social determinants are multiplied across the lifespan. Action taken throughout the lifespan could both provide opportunities for those with poor mental health and greatly reduce the occurrence of certain mental disorders. As mental health is inextricably linked to physical health, these interventions could also improve physical health and enhance overall health.

Figure 5.1: A life course approach to tackling inequalities in health

Broad themes

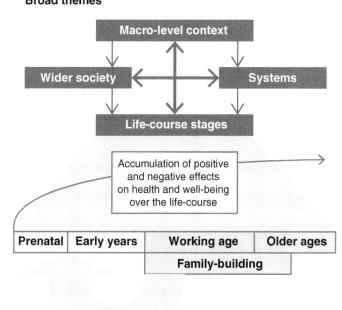

Source: reproduced from WHO (2014c, p xv)

The WHO review of the social determinants of mental health (WHO, 2008) took a life course perspective (see Figure 5.1), demonstrating that influences at different stages of life can have profound impacts on mental health. The WHO argue that it is particularly important that action is taken early in the life course and that this continues through to older age. This approach provides the support required to ensure that people are given the chance to flourish. Interventions during these different life stages can both improve mental health and reduce the impact of wider social inequalities.

Based on their review of the factors influencing mental health, Lund et al (2018) stress that there is a wide range of determinants and many of these present measurement challenges. They conceptualise social determinants across five domains:

- demographic
- social
- economic
- neighbourhood
- environmental events

These are then further broken down into distal (upstream, indirectly affecting health) and proximal (downstream, directly affecting health) factors, which interact in complex and complicated ways.

Some of the key social determinants of mental health are discussed next.

Age

Ageism is an invisible and pervasive form of discrimination that involves prejudice against people because of their age. Like racism and sexism, ageism invokes negative stereotypes about people. While it is important to remember that ageism affects both young and old people, the stigma against mental health disorders is greater in later life. Ageism results in a range of harms, disadvantages and injustices, including reduced life expectancy and poorer health outcomes. The WHO suggest ageism is a global problem that contributes to poor outcomes, including social isolation, premature death and high economic costs. In the *Global Report on Ageism*, they note: 'Often people fail to recognize the existence of such institutional ageism because the rules, norms and practices of the institution are of long-standing, have become ritualized and are seen as normal' (WHO, 2021a, p 5).

Ageing is often discussed by the general public and the media using negative stereotypes based on declining mental and cognitive functions. This pejorative view of later life may be internalised and enacted by older individuals themselves, creating a vicious circle that worsens mental health. Ageism is a global issue which permeates most sectors of society, including education, employment and health and social care. The WHO call for urgent action on this 'insidious' scourge on society (WHO, 2021a). They estimate that, worldwide, approximately 6.3 million cases of depression are attributable to ageism (WHO, 2021a). In healthcare, rationing based on age is commonplace. The WHO report recommends three concrete actions that all stakeholders can take to combat ageism: 'invest in evidence-based strategies to prevent and tackle ageism'; 'improve data and research to gain a better understanding of ageism and how to reduce it'; and 'build a movement to change the narrative around age and ageing' (WHO, 2021a, p xvii).

A systemic review revealed that in 85 per cent of 149 studies, age determined who received certain medical procedures (Chang et al, 2020). Age bias can devalue older people's lives and negatively affect the level and nature of care they receive. Combating ageism is one of the four action areas for the Decade of Healthy Ageing (2021–30) declared by the United Nations and the WHO. However, Mikton et al (2021) argue that the Decade of Healthy Ageing can only become a reality if ageism is recognised and tackled as a social determinant of health.

The COVID-19 pandemic exposed the extent of ageism in a wide range of settings, including healthcare, the media and economic structures, highlighting the vulnerability of older people. Media portrayals of older people as a burden and social media hashtags such as #BoomerRemover demonstrated how different generations can be pitted against each other. Older people were widely misrepresented and undervalued in the discourse surrounding the pandemic. In some instances, the pandemic was depicted as a problem for older people rather than for society as a whole. Prejudices against, and stereotypes about, older people are associated with depression and self-stigma. Older people may neglect their physical and mental wellbeing as they internalise ideas that they are less valuable.

Childhood is a crucial period of development and growth: it plays a critical role in shaping later life. Adverse conditions in early life are associated with higher risks of mental disorders. Family circumstances and the quality of parenting have a significant impact on the risk of poor mental and physical health. Early experiences lay the foundations for robust mental health. If children live in difficult circumstances, or are exposed to adverse conditions, this can have negative short- and long-term consequences. Disruptions to the developmental process can have lifelong implications (see Figure 5.2).

The critical nature of the parent and child interaction has been stressed by University College London's Institute of Health Equity; it noted that 'lack of secure attachment, lack of quality stimulation within and outside the home, and conflict ... negatively impact on future social behaviour, educational outcomes, employment status and health' (Bell et al, 2013, pp 24–5). Children's exposure to neglect, direct physical and psychological abuse, and growing up in families with domestic violence were particularly damaging. Parental mental health plays a key role in outcomes for children. For example, children of mothers with mental ill health are five times more likely to have mental disorders (Melzer et al, 2003). Poverty, and particularly debt, can increase maternal stress. Exposure to multiple risks is particularly damaging, as effects accumulate. However, impact can be offset by protective parenting activities, such as good social and emotional interactions. These inequalities in early years' development are potentially remediable through family and parenting support, maternal care, childcare and education. Wider family and strong communities can also act as buffers and sources of support to ameliorate impact. For adolescents, education is essential for fostering emotional resilience, which could act as a buffer to poor outcomes in later life.

Education

Education and health, including mental health, are inextricably linked. There is a wealth of compelling evidence to suggest that education is one of the most significant social determinants of health (The Lancet Global Health, 2020). Education shapes lives and is positively correlated with life expectancy, morbidity and health behaviours. It plays a key role in health by shaping opportunities for employment and income. A large-scale study (Wu et al, 2020) found that the differences in education and wealth established at an early stage in life were strongly associated with differences in

Figure 5.2: Experience of mental health issues across the life course

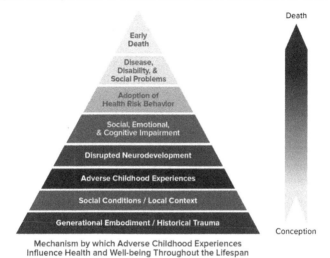

Mechanism by which Adverse Childhood Experiences
Influence Health and Well-being Throughout the Lifespan

Source: CDC (2022)

healthy ageing. Across the life cycle, low education led to persistent disadvantage in terms of health outcomes. Work by Parker et al (2020) also illustrates the lifelong impact of education on healthy ageing. Their study examined healthy working life expectancy at age 50 in England and highlighted that inequalities were linked to educational attainment. Poor attainment was associated with insecure employment, manual labour, poor working conditions and uncertainty. Longer healthy working life expectancy was linked to access to opportunities.

Education is a way out of poverty: it can reduce socioeconomic and health inequalities. In recent years, the centrality of education to good mental health has become much more apparent. Fundamentally, a good-quality education supports the development of a child's emotional, cognitive and communication skills. Individuals can learn about forming relationships and psychological wellbeing. It equips children with the ability to cope with stress, self-regulate emotional challenges, understand and manage their own mental health and nurture others. Education provides the basis for forming relationships and understanding social norms and values. Gnanapragasam et al (2023) highlight that education at all levels is crucial, noting that literacy in language supports emotional literacy. Rates of smoking, obesity, cervical cancer and depression have been found to be higher in those with the lowest levels of formal education (Alder and Rehkopf, 2008; Powers, 2015). Poverty, poor housing, deprivation, inequality, low self-esteem and insecure employment are intertwined.

Education is a critical social determinant of health largely because of its substantial impact on other social determinants. Poor education is a key social determinant of poor mental health, including the risk of mental illnesses and substance use disorders, as well as worsening outcomes for individuals affected by these disorders (Compton and Shim, 2015). Not only does education give individuals a chance of upward mobility, placing them in better financial circumstances to access quality healthcare, but it also keeps them better informed of how to take care of their health.

The adverse impact of poor education on mental health relates to a number of key issues, described next.

Reduced stress

Better-educated individuals are likely to receive higher incomes and will often have lower levels of the health-harming stresses associated with prolonged social and economic hardship. Lower levels of educational attainment are associated with fewer resources, not just financial resources, but also the social support, sense of control over life and self-esteem that can buffer the effects of stress. Life events that cause trauma, chronic anxiety and discrimination can lead to health-harming stress. Economic hardship and other stressors can have a cumulative negative effect on health over time and may, in turn, make individuals more sensitive to further stressors. Researchers have coined the term 'allostatic load' to refer to the effects of chronic exposure to physiological stress responses. Exposure to high allostatic load over time may predispose individuals to illnesses such as asthma, cardiovascular disease, gastrointestinal disease and infections, all associated with higher death rates among older adults (Parker et al, 2022).

Social and psychological skills

Formal education in school (alongside learning opportunities outside the classroom) builds skills and fosters traits that are important throughout life, such as conscientiousness, perseverance, a sense of personal control, flexibility, the capacity for negotiation and the ability to form relationships and establish social networks. These skills are essential to address many of the challenges posed throughout the life cycle, such as maintaining a good work-life balance, managing one's own emotional and physical health and navigating the labyrinthine healthcare system. Through education, a broad spectrum of skills can be developed, including problem-solving, and key personality traits can be fostered. Education can increase 'learned effectiveness', improving cognitive ability, self-control and problem-solving. Personality traits, otherwise known as 'soft skills', are associated with success in education and employment, and they lead to lower mortality rates. One set of these personality traits has been called the 'Big Five': conscientiousness; openness to experience; being extraverted; being agreeable; and emotional stability (Power, 2015). By enhancing these various forms of human capital, education can affect health. For example, education may strengthen 'coping skills' that reduce the damage of stress. Greater personal control may also lead to healthier behaviours, partly by increasing knowledge. Those with greater perceived personal control are more associated with preventive behaviours.

Social networks

Educated adults tend to have larger social networks – and these connections produce access to financial, psychological and emotional resources that may help reduce hardship and stress, while improving health. Social networks enhance access to information and exposure to peers who model acceptable behaviours. The relationship between social support and education may be due, in part, to social and cognitive skills and the fact that civic participation increases with more education. Years of political science research suggest that education has a universally positive impact on all forms of civil engagement (Campbell, 2009). Low social support is associated with higher death rates and poor mental health. Social support plays a crucial role in maintaining and promoting health, and its absence is a major factor where there is a higher incidence of poor mental health.

Knowledge and skills

In addition to being prepared for better jobs, people with more education are much more likely to be informed about healthy behaviours. Educated individuals may be better able to understand their health needs, follow instructions, advocate for themselves and their families, and communicate effectively with health providers. They are more likely to seek help at an early stage and engage in health-promoting activities, such as physical exercise.

Ethnicity

Racism, exclusion and alienation experienced by members of ethnic minorities increase risks for a range of mental disorders. Experiencing racism can be extremely stressful and negatively impact an individual's mental health. According to the Mental Health Foundation (2023), exposure to racism may increase the likelihood of mental health problems such as psychosis and depression. In a large case-control study of cumulative social disadvantage, ethnicity and first-episode psychosis in the UK, there was a clear linear association between cumulative disadvantage and the odds of psychosis, with Black Caribbeans experiencing greater social disadvantage and isolation than White British subjects (Morgan et al, 2008). Institutional racism results in poorer-quality treatment and ethnic differences in pathways to care. There is evidence that living in an area with few of one's own ethnic group is a risk factor for psychosis. This may be partly explained by the lack of social support, which could have been protective (Schofield et al, 2023).

Research by the Race Equality Foundation in 2022 highlights a range of issues associated with the unequal outcomes and life chances of diverse communities. They criticise the government for not focusing on the inequalities in accessing mental health services for Black, Asian and other ethnic minority communities. The significant flaws in the system meant that it was not fit for purpose. The report stresses that racial inequality remains a major problem in UK mental health services (Race Equality Foundation, 2022). The COVID-19 pandemic shone a spotlight on these long-standing inequalities, highlighting the mismatch between the needs of those seeking mental health support and the services available. The report stresses that many Black communities were struggling to navigate a patchy mental health pathway.

Gender

Globally, it is well established that women are at greater risk of developing common mental disorders, such as depression, whereas men are at higher risk of substance misuse (Albert, 2015). The effects of gender are frequently interconnected with other social determinants of mental health. Gender affects not only the prevalence of disorders, but also the risk, timing, diagnosis, treatment and response to poor mental health.

The social construction of gender identity and the unequal power relations between men and women affect mental health outcomes. Women's mental health cannot be viewed in isolation from their broader role in society. This role is characterised by social inequality, which affects the types of mental health issues women experience and how these are framed by society and health professionals. Any discussion of social determinants needs to include how gender norms around motherhood, family life, caring roles and economic activity create an increased burden on women. Gender and feminist discourses have emerged as a significant framework for examining determinants of mental health. Many aspects of life – such as access to resources, cultural expectations, ambition, competitiveness, social roles and responsibility – are thought to be linked to higher prevalence of psychological disorders.

The most common forms of violence against women – domestic abuse and sexual abuse – contribute significantly to women's stress and increased risk of mental ill health. It has been estimated that 35 per cent of women worldwide have experienced partner violence or non-partner sexual violence. According to the WHO (WHO et al, 2013), women are significantly more likely than men to have experienced severe violence. Globally, almost 39 per cent of murders of women are committed by sexual partners or ex-partners (compared to 10 per cent of men; Garcia-Vergara et al, 2022). Power inequalities mean that domestic violence, including physical attacks, coercive control and intimidation, disproportionately affect women. These factors are likely to have a negative impact on women's behaviour in relation to their health and may explain why treatment plans are not adhered to and prescribed medications are not taken.

As part of the socialisation process, young boys become aware of the acceptable male traits, including assertiveness, toughness, domination, confidence, being unemotional and ambition. Characteristics such as vulnerability, emotional awareness, demonstrating affection and passiveness are associated with females and are therefore to be avoided. Men should be protectors, leaders, breadwinners. These outdated but prevalent stereotypes underpin gender socialisation and affect behaviours, creating an unhealthy understanding of what gender means in today's society. Perpetuating these ideas can mean that individuals harm themselves and others.

Other structural inequalities intersect with poor mental health and increase the risks for women. For example, low income and low levels of education make it more likely that women who suffer domestic violence will remain in abusive relationships. Poor women are particularly at risk of common mental disorders and, conversely, women with poor mental health are particularly vulnerable to higher levels of poverty.

Economic circumstances

There is an indisputable link between economic inequality and poor mental health. (Saraceno et al, 1997). Poverty is a key driver of poor mental health. One of the most insidious effects of poverty is the psychological stress it imposes. (As already noted, the social gradient in mental health means that higher levels of poverty are linked to a higher prevalence of mental illnesses, such as schizophrenia.) Socioeconomic disadvantage, unemployment, debt and social exclusion are consistently associated with mental health problems. Social marginalisation, discrimination and economic disadvantage have powerful effects on mental health. Individuals are made vulnerable to mental ill health through poverty, social inequality and discrimination. In their research, Campo-Arias et al (2021) used social stress theory to explain the relationship between poverty and poor mental health. People in socially disadvantaged situations have more stressors and increased vulnerability to stress due to scarce psychosocial resources, leading to higher risk of psychological distress or mental disorder.

Poverty is both a cause of mental illness and a consequence (Knifton and Inglis, 2020). It is a two-way street. Poverty increases the risk of mental illness, including depression and schizophrenia, while having a serious mental illness can result in a lower socioeconomic status. Mental health problems can lead to difficulties in securing and retaining employment and to underemployment. This vicious cycle is complex, leading to relatively high levels of mental illness among people living in the most deprived circumstances. Poverty is associated with high levels of stress. Some people move in and out of poverty, but persistent poverty is associated with the worst mental health outcomes. Predictably, poverty and financial insecurity are significant risk factors for a wide range of psychological illnesses. Poverty takes a heavy toll on individuals' mental health, leaving them with a reduced ability to deal with everyday stresses and strains.

Poverty is particularly harmful for children. Children in lower socioeconomic groups are less likely to experience conditions that facilitate optimal development. Exposure to stress from poor economic circumstances can permanently affect cognitive development. Poverty in childhood can cause a lack of resilience and an inability to address life stresses. Exposure to poverty at an early age can have a lasting negative impact on health, with increased susceptibility to certain cancers and cardiac disease (Fell and Hewstone, 2015). Being raised in environments of low socioeconomic status is associated with lower educational attainment and poorer cognitive performance, particularly in the area of language development. Social and emotional difficulties related to social gradients have been shown among children as young as 3 years. Analysis from the UK found that family income was inversely related to socio-emotional difficulties in children (Allen et al, 2014). Poverty is associated with negative stereotypes, including labels such as 'scrounger' and 'workshy'. These perceptions can lead to self-stigma and affect belief in the ability to succeed. The debilitating impact of deprivation is toxic to children.

Stable and appropriately remunerated employment is the key to many social determinants of health. The financial stability it provides can enable individuals to live in safer neighbourhoods, afford better healthcare, provide education or childcare for their children and buy nutritious food. Unemployment and underemployment place strain on financial resources and are barriers to meeting basic needs. Unemployed individuals are likely to self-report worse health status, may experience more depressive symptoms and are at higher risk of premature mortality. Employment is strongly associated with reduced symptoms of depression and anxiety as well as lower prevalence of suicide, especially among men. Employment is an important protective factor against mental disorders, and it is associated with better social functioning, less severe symptoms, better quality of life and improved self-esteem in people living with schizophrenia and bipolar disorder (Lund et al, 2018).

There is an extensive body of evidence illustrating the devastating effects of economic recession on individual and community mental health. Following the 2008 global financial crisis, research showed that unemployment and insecure employment were key contributors to an increase in depression (Campo-Arias and De Mendieta, 2021). The stress associated with precarious employment and lack of financial security also contributed to increased rates of self-harm and suicide. Following the 2008 financial crisis, cases of self-harm and suicide increased dramatically in the Republic of Ireland (Corcoran et al, 2015). Vulnerable groups without a financial cushion are hardest hit by a deterioration in labour markets. Levels of poverty and social exclusion worsen mainly in groups that were already dealing with financial disadvantage. The global post-pandemic cost of living crisis has been particularly challenging for low-income households, with increased stress and anxiety about being unable to pay bills or buy food. The Mental Health Foundation (2023) has predicted that the effects of the cost-of-living crisis in the UK will be on a scale similar to the effects of the COVID-19 pandemic. Poverty and financial stress are associated with a cycle of worry and anxiety. Concerns about money impinge on people's ability to engage in activities that have a protective impact on their mental wellbeing.

Neighbourhood

In recent years, there has been a growing awareness of the significance of place and space on mental health. The neighbourhoods that people live in comprise their homes, the places where they work and socialise and the built environment between these. The built environment has both direct and indirect impacts on mental health, which can be due to air quality, water quality, noise and traffic. High-quality places, spaces and buildings encourage people to be more physically active, feel safe and secure, use facilities and services, and socialise and play. For example, well-maintained and accessible green spaces facilitate physical activity. It has been estimated that on average people spend around 90 per cent of their time indoors, with the majority of this being within the home (Mannan et al, 2021). Numerous housing-related factors are associated with mental and physical health impacts. These include condensation, dampness, infestation, noise, lighting, housing tenure and housing design. For example, higher residential density interferes with the development of socially supportive relationships within the household (Barros et al, 2019). For optimal health, individuals require well-designed homes that are insulated, warm and have enough space to meet their needs. Overcrowding can lead to stress and family violence, including child maltreatment, intimate partner violence, sexual violence and abuse of older people.

The WHO (2008) identified the five main indoor air substances that have a detrimental effect as being radon, tobacco smoke, cooking pollutants, volatile organic compounds and asbestos, all of which are linked to respiratory diseases. In the UK, outdoor air quality is largely affected by traffic, solid fuel burning and industrial pollutants. Exposure to harmful pollutants and toxins have a deleterious impact on physical and mental health. Children exposed to significant air pollution are at higher risk of delayed brain development and debilitating respiratory conditions, as well as cancers and strokes, as adults.

Noise-related problems are more prevalent in areas of high socioeconomic need and are associated with disturbed sleep, resulting in poor mental health. Homes that are insulated from noise and peaceful can support the wellbeing of their residents.

In addition to direct effects, the built environment can indirectly impact mental health by impinging on social cohesion and community development. Social networks can act as essential social support systems to protect mental health and act as buffers against stress. These networks are linked to better health practices, such as enhanced self-management and reduced use of health services.

Social connectedness is the degree to which people have the desired number, quality and diversity of relationships to sustain a sense of value and belonging. The amount and quality of relationships matter: close bonds create a sense of security. They are important for the wellbeing and recovery of people with mental illness, who are more likely to have difficulty forming and maintaining relationships. Human beings are social creatures and connections are highly valued. Social connectedness and belonging can help to create trust and resilience within communities. A sense of community engenders hope and can improve the ability to recover from stress, depression and anxiety.

There is a wealth of evidence (Sintonen and Pehkonen, 2014; Newan and Zainal, 2020) showing that satisfying relationships and friendships are fundamental to wellbeing. Social connection is a protective factor against depression, sleep problems and dementia, including Alzheimer's disease. The beneficial effects of social networks and social support have been well established in a multitude of studies (see Saphire-Berstein and Taylor, 2013). Having a close family and support network has been consistently shown to be associated with better mental health and wellbeing.

Conversely, loneliness and social isolation can have serious consequences for the physical and mental health of individuals. Lonely people are more likely to be depressed, less satisfied, less happy and more pessimistic. A lack of social support is associated with depression, emotional distress and poor psychological functioning. Loneliness is a key indicator of impaired social wellbeing (Lincoln, 2000; Mushtag et al, 2014). It is associated with a loss of cognition in older age. According to the 2021 UK Census, loneliness affects almost a quarter of the UK population. Many studies have demonstrated the link between loneliness and poor mental outcomes, including depression, anxiety and psychosis. The stress-buffering model (Folkman and Lazarus, 1986) demonstrates the role that social support plays in buffering the impact of loneliness and depressive symptoms. Contrary to popular opinion, older people are not the loneliest group in the population – young children and adolescents report the highest levels of loneliness. It has been suggested by Mushtag et al (2014) that this phenomenon can be explained by older people having better developed coping skills and lower expectations than younger people. Loneliness is associated with a loss of cognition and perceptual awareness. It has been suggested that loneliness is associated with a twofold increased risk of dementia, with some authors proposing that it represents an early stage of dementia (Holwerda, 2012).

Environmental events

Negative life events that occur as a result of natural disasters, war and conflict have been identified as strong determinants of mental illness. War is a common feature of our world. The United Nations (2019) estimates that nearly 132 million people in 42 countries around the world needed humanitarian assistance resulting from conflict or disaster in 2019. Nearly 69 million people worldwide had been forcibly displaced by violence and conflict, the highest number since World War Two. The WHO estimate that in areas affected by conflict, one in five people are living with a mental disorder and one in ten are living with a moderate or severe mental disorder. Many studies have revealed that children exposed to armed conflict are at risk of a range of negative outcomes, including heightened aggression, anxiety, depression and post-traumatic stress disorder (PTSD; Bogic et al, 2015; Bratti et al, 2015; World Bank, 2016; McDonald, 2017).

Extensive research has concluded that the prolonged civil conflict in Northern Ireland (known as 'the Troubles'), in which 3,500 people died and 47,000 were seriously injured, had an adverse impact on the mental health of the citizens (Kelleher, 2003; Ferry et al, 2010; Ulster University, 2015). In 2008, 39 per cent of the population in Northern Ireland reported they had experienced a traumatic event relating to the Troubles (Bunting et al, 2012). One in five adults experienced a mental health problem, a rate that was 25 per cent higher than in England. Prior to the pandemic, one in eight children had emotional difficulties. A study in 2011 found that Northern Ireland had the highest recorded rate of PTSD of any studied country in the world (Ferry et al, 2011). It continues to have one of the highest rates of suicide in the UK and Ireland (O'Neill et al, 2019). Northern Ireland also has the highest level of maternal mental health problems in the UK (O'Neill et al, 2019).

A major study of the consequences of the Troubles (Bamford Centre for Mental Health and Wellbeing, 2011) shed considerable light on the relationship between trauma and poor mental health. Individuals who experienced any conflict-related traumatic event were more likely to have developed a lifelong anxiety, mood swings, substance misuse or impulse control disorder compared to those who experienced a non-conflict-related traumatic event and those who had not experienced a traumatic event. The transgenerational impact of the Troubles in Northern Ireland is increasingly a focus for many researchers and clinicians, with some estimating that potentially 60 per cent of the adult population with mental health problems directly linked to the Troubles have not received support. It is argued that to help those affected by the transmission of trauma, an understanding of the ways in which trauma is transmitted is imperative. Despite the prevalence of poor mental health, the level of public spending on this area is markedly lower in Northern Ireland than in the rest of the UK. In England in 2019, some 12 per cent of the overall health budget was spent on mental health, compared with 6 per cent in Northern Ireland.

Research has highlighted the extent to which the COVID-19 pandemic can be viewed as a major traumatic event for individuals and communities. In many ways, the impact has been similar to that from previous infectious disease epidemics. The social determinants of mental health had a profound impact on this trauma. Ettman et al (2020) found that poverty, discrimination and job insecurity were exacerbated for many families and communities during the COVID-19 pandemic, contributing to trauma. Any government preparation for a further global public health emergency must address the social determinants of health inequalities. The COVID-19 pandemic has brought into sharp focus the inequalities that already existed globally in terms of gender, ethnic origin, socioeconomic status and migratory status and how these acted as mediators and moderators of the mental health impact of the pandemic.

Conclusion

In recent decades in the field of mental health, research attention has been drawn increasingly to the social determinants of health – the factors apart from medical care that can be influenced by social policies and shape health in powerful ways. There is a broad acceptance that because mental disorders are so strongly socially determined, the global burden of these disorders will not be relieved by improved access to mental health treatments alone. Social and genetic causes of disease are no longer viewed as mutually exclusive. For example, neighbourhood-level socioeconomic deprivation is associated with an increased risk of psychotic disorders. Individuals living in neighbourhoods associated with poverty have fewer sources of support to address vulnerability. The idea that poor mental health can simply be explained by 'faulty wiring' or a 'bad gene' has been debunked. The social and political context is as important, if not more important, than individual characteristics or genetics. We now know the important role played by social and physical environments and how social and public policies can mitigate the impact of these contextual factors.

Social policies and institutions – in education, social care, healthcare and work – also have a marked impact on mental health, for better or worse. To reduce inequities and promote good mental health, it is vital that action is taken to enhance the conditions of life across the life cycle, beginning before birth and progressing into early childhood, older childhood and adolescence, family-building and working years and older age. Therefore, mental health policy must be comprehensive and multidisciplinary. Interventions should not be done to communities, but with communities. Co-producing effective policies which empower individuals and communities should underpin interventions on social determinants.

Further reading

Compton, M.T. and Shim, R.S. (eds) (2015) *The Social Determinants of Mental Health*, Washington, DC: American Psychiatric Association.
Marmot, M. and Wilkinson, R. (eds) (2005) *Social Determinants of Health* (2nd edn) Oxford: Oxford University Press.

6

Stigma

Introduction

Stigma is complex and prevalent. It is based on a set of negative beliefs that an individual or a society has about something or someone. People with mental disorders have been stigmatised for centuries in different countries and cultures. More than any other types of illness, negative judgements are associated with mental disorders. The most prominent stereotypes surrounding mental illness presume unpredictability, dangerousness and violence – ideas that have been perpetuated by misleading media reports. The pernicious impact of stigma on the lives of people with mental illness is hard to overstate. Among other things, it influences self-belief, help-seeking behaviours and public and professional responses. This chapter discusses the concept of stigma, identifies types of stigma, outlines the importance of language, discusses the concept of toxic masculinity and assesses a number of interventions designed to address the issue of stigma and mental health.

Nature of stigma

The Oxford English Dictionary (2022) defines stigma as a mark or sign of disgrace or discredit. The word 'stigmatisation' indicates negative connotations: in ancient Greece, a 'stigma' was a brand to mark slaves or criminals (Rössler, 2016). Stigma is used to discredit or marginalise those who are deemed to be different from others in a society, and stigmatisation of the mentally ill has a very long history.

There is no country, society or culture in the world where individuals with a mental illness have the same value as people without a mental illness (Rössler, 2016).

For centuries, mental illness was regarded as a punishment from God. Sufferers were believed to be possessed by evil spirits and were punished, tortured and killed. The women who were burnt as witches in Europe and North America in the 16th and 17th centuries are now widely believed to have been suffering from mental illness. In the 19th century, 'lunatic asylums' and 'madhouses' were built to detain individuals, often far away from their local communities. Ideas of evil spirits or demons possessing people and influencing their behaviour were used in many cultures to justify erratic behaviour or explain symptoms.

Highly vulnerable people were subject to the most extraordinary behaviours to 'evict' or break the stronghold of these demons. As Rogers and Pilgrim (2003, p 5) point out: 'Unlike those with physical impairments or the old and frail, the mad were also feared and distrusted. Consequently, treatments viewed as "scandalous" when imposed on the sane have been deemed to be acceptable, both legally and ethically, for the "insane."'

In his seminal 1963 book *Stigma: Notes on the Management of Spoiled Identity*, sociologist Erving Goffman set a new course for understanding stigma as a socially constructed concept existing in the relationship between a discredited attribute and the audience receiving the attribute. He outlines the position of the 'discredited' within society in the early 1960s, referring to stigmatised individuals as 'reduced from a whole and usual person to a tainted discounted one' (Goffman, 1963, p 12). He distinguishes between 'normals' and discredited individuals (p 15). For Goffman, stigma is a general aspect of social life that complicates everyday micro-level interactions. The stigmatised may be wary of engaging with those who do not share their stigma, and those without a certain stigma may disparage, overcompensate for or attempt to ignore stigmatised individuals. Developing Goffman's work, Link and Phelan (2001) suggest that stigma exists only in the presence of additional factors, such as 'othering' – the separation of 'them' from 'us', with 'us' holding power over 'them'. They examine the issue from a broad socio-structural view and contend that stigma exists when the following key elements are present:

- People must be able to identify and label a certain social trait or difference (such as mental illness) as socially significant. This results in culturally derived categories that are used to differentiate people into groups.
- These differences are labelled as undesirable, therefore creating a negative cultural stereotype that is applied to this group.
- Those who are labelled are perceived to be significantly different, thereby creating the idea of 'them' and 'us'.
- Stigmatised groups are socially devalued, disparaged and disadvantaged in terms of access to key social determinants, such as health, housing, education and employment. Discrimination occurs at both a structural and an individual level.
- Discrimination is completely dependent on access to social and economic power, as only those who have power can disadvantage and marginalise others.

While the concept of stigma has evolved since Goffman first introduced his theory, his ideas have endured and are often cited in academic work on the topic. The subject has developed and grown into a significant area of research within the social science arena, and it is of crucial importance for better understanding of mental health discourses.

It is generally accepted that stigma can have far-reaching consequences for individuals, families and society. Perceptions of dangerous and unpredictable behaviours related to mental illness have led to societal fear and distrust, giving rise to discrimination that is felt in the lives of many of those affected by mental illness (Mannarini and Rossi, 2019). There are also significant differences in stigmatisation depending on the type of disorder. Schizophrenia is more likely to be associated with negative attitudes than depression or anxiety. People with mental illness are more likely to be rejected by employers and landlords, and more likely to experience poverty (Jenkins et al, 2008). Corrigan (2018) suggests that attempts to define mental health stigma must contend with three competing agendas: the services agenda, which focuses on avoiding labels to encourage engagement in services; the rights-based agenda, which aims to minimise negative depictions of mental illness; and the self-worth agenda, which stresses the importance of encouraging self-worth and pride among people who are experiencing mental distress.

It is important to note that stigma around mental illness reinforces other forms of stigma, such as those based on disability, gender, race, poverty and sexuality. The impact of this interaction leads to disproportionately high rates of diagnosis of mental illness among certain groups of people – for example, African American people are more likely than White people to have a diagnosis. Recent research has emphasised the significance of intersectional stigma to explain the convergence of multiple stigmatised identities. Put simply, multiple disadvantages increase the likelihood of poor mental health and magnify its impact on an individual's life. The reality is that you are much more likely to experience poor mental health if you are living in poverty. And if you do, then you will likely experience more stigma and discrimination. Its impact on your life – on education, employment, housing and health, for example – will be greater, and it will be more difficult to recover from. Stigma is a significant cause of social disadvantage and inextricably linked to health inequalities. It can impact negatively on a range of life chances and on a multitude of outcomes. Mental illness stigma intersects with other marginalising factors and results in adverse consequences.

Social psychologists suggest that stigma is manifested in individual internalisation and ensuing behavioural processes that connect to interrelated components, such as stereotypes, labelling, discrimination and power imbalances (Rusch et al, 2005). Stereotypes are explained by Corrigan and Bink (2016) as perceived factual knowledge structures that are inherent in cultures with associated negative connotations. The idea that people who have mental ill health are somehow responsible for their illness is a commonly heard injurious, powerful stereotype which Weiner (1995) explains in terms of onset and offset responsibility: onset responsibility occurs when the blamed individual incurs a condition through exposure and absorption of the mental illness; and offset responsibility suggests a person is responsible for their condition because they have not engaged in suitable treatment for recovery.

An especially damaging stereotype is the belief that individuals with a mental health condition possess dangerous and criminal tendencies; this idea is applied to people with schizophrenia and bipolar disorder in particular (Corrigan and Bink, 2016). The resulting fear leads to more precarious inequitable practices, including avoidance and withdrawal. Fear of being physically or verbally assaulted leads members of the public to avoid individuals with a mental disorder. This may explain why people tend to react negatively when mental health support provisions relocate in their immediate vicinity (Corrigan and Bink, 2016). This labelling and stereotyping process gives rise to separation of groups. Society does not want to be associated with unattractive characteristics, and thus hierarchical categories are created. Once these categories develop, the groups who have the most undesirable characteristics may experience status loss and discrimination. The entire process is accompanied by significant embarrassment on the part of the individuals themselves and those associated with them (Link and Phelan, 2001).

Over the past century, society has come a long way in terms of our knowledge and understanding of mental health issues. Yet in many ways, our attitudes and perceptions are still outdated and discriminatory. Mental health-related discrimination and stigma are global, complex problems. Henderson and Gronholm (2018) argue that mental health-related stigma should be considered a 'wicked problem'. This would enable a broader understanding of the concept and facilitate a wide range of interventions. The Mental Health Foundation (2022) estimates that almost nine out of ten people who suffer from a mental health problem experience stigma at some point in their lives. The WHO states that 'the most important barrier to overcome in the community is stigma and discrimination towards people with a mental health or behavioural disorder' (2021, p 98).

Stigma can maintain discrimination and marginalisation and reduce empathy and understanding. In their analysis of the social perception of mental and physical health conditions, Robinson et al (2019) found that compared to physical health conditions, mental health conditions were more likely to be stigmatised and trivialised. The results varied by condition, with schizophrenia the most stigmatised and obsessive-compulsive disorder the most trivialised. Many individuals not only have to cope with the often devastating effects of their illness, but also suffer from social exclusion because of ignorance and fear. Some people describe the shame and ostracisation associated with stigma as worse than the condition itself (Thornicroft et al, 2016).

As well as discrimination based on stigma, people with a mental illness are more likely to experience poverty and have limited life chances. This combination of illness, oppression and marginalisation is hugely detrimental to self-esteem and self-efficacy. The impact of a mental illness diagnosis, and the consequent labelling and discrimination associated with this, will have a detrimental impact on an individual already experiencing the negative effects of living on the margins. Ideas of stigma, prejudice, stereotypes, labelling and othering are closely linked, robustly debated and contested across a wide range of disciplines.

While things have improved markedly since the late 1990s, mental illness remains shrouded in mystery and plagued by myths and misconceptions. Despite the overall prevalence of mental illness, increasing numbers of people needing mental health treatment do not receive it. Stigma has been identified as a significant barrier to seeking and obtaining help. Due to the stigma of mental illness, '61% fear seeking help for a mental health problem' (Rethink Mental Illness, 2021).

Types of stigma

Different types of stigma have been identified (see Corrigan and Watson, 2002; Subu et al, 2021):

- Public stigma – this refers to the negative attitudes held by members of the public about those with mental illnesses.

- Self-stigma – this refers to the negative attitudes, including internalised shame, that people with mental illness have about their own condition.
- Institutional stigma – this is more systemic, involving policies of organisations that intentionally or unintentionally limit opportunities for people with mental illness.

Public stigma

Public stigma is a process by which the general public and society endorse the negative stereotypes associated with mental illness and subsequently participate in prejudicial and discriminatory practices (Corrigan, 2004, 2008; Corrigan et al, 2016). The behavioural aspect of public stigma includes avoidance, evasion, coercive treatment and social segregation.

In their review of the medical literature on stigma and public attitudes towards mental illness, Hayward and Bright (1997) found four themes:

- Dangerousness – there was a commonplace perception that people with a mental illness are dangerous, unpredictable and violent.
- Attribute of responsibility – there was a perception that individuals are responsible for their own poor mental health. This was linked to their lifestyle or life choices.
- Poor prognosis – this concerns the perception that there is little or any hope of recovery from a mental illness; it is a life sentence, something that could not be 'cured' or successfully treated.
- Disruption of social interaction – this relates to the perception that the cause of stigma lies in the disruption of norms about social roles.

By labelling people with a mental illness, the public emphasises and reinforces their deviation from societal standards and norms. Rather than encounter damaging and difficult social interactions, sufferers withdraw from social interactions, thereby reducing their participation in society and everyday life. This isolation and social retreat diminishes self-esteem and, in turn, increases vulnerability to psychosocial stress. Consequently, the social networks of those with a mental illness are often relatively small and restricted.

Self-stigma

Self-stigma can result in pernicious outcomes for health and wellbeing. Self-stigma is associated with a range of negative outcomes, including increased depression, social avoidance, decreased self-esteem, worsening psychological distress and decreased help seeking. These negative emotional reactions limit access to support and treatment. Internalised stigma is an impediment to recovery and adds to the burden of poor mental health (Corrigan and Rao, 2012). There is extensive evidence supporting the link between poor self-image and reduced help seeking (Lannin and Bible, 2022). This acts as a barrier to recovery and is likely to worsen symptoms and magnify the overall impact of the illness.

Self-stigma in the form of withdrawal from society or decreased use of healthcare services results in reduced quality of life. Low self-esteem and limited confidence can also lead to decisions not to avail of opportunities related to education and employment, thereby reducing the likelihood of living an independent life. Setting goals and having personal ambition is viewed as a waste of time, as 'normal' outcomes are unattainable. Research consistently indicates that self-stigma and public stigma have the most influence over help-seeking for mental illness. It acts as a barrier to individuals seeking help, as they experience feelings of low self-esteem, shame and embarrassment and an unwillingness to disclose their weakness.

Not seeking or pursuing treatment results in social isolation, marginalisation and feelings of hopelessness. The outcome of self-stigmatisation may be that people feel trapped in a cycle of illness with nowhere to turn or no means to escape. Feelings of shame and embarrassment among young people mean they may withdraw from society, develop negative perceptions about paid employment and not pursue careers or educational opportunities.

Stereotype agreement refers to individuals affirming and internalising the perceived negative beliefs of the public (Corrigan et al, 2011). Self-concurrence occurs when the individual believes those negative stereotypes that are applied to them, leading to diminishing self-esteem and self-efficacy (Corrigan et al, 2011). Individuals can become resigned to not trying to achieve personal goals, as described by Corrigan et al (2009) as the 'why try' effect: There is no point in applying for this job – no one will employ someone like me. This process is illustrated in Figure 6.1.

Institutional stigma

Institutional stigma around mental health refers to an institution (a government, company or school, for instance) having policies or a culture based on negative attitudes and beliefs about people with mental health problems. For instance, Corrigan and Shapiro (2010) assert that discrimination in employment and housing is more likely to occur for those with a mental illness than those without. Structural stigma is where stigmatised beliefs are held by a large part of a society. Stigma is embedded in the social framework, and this creates perceptions about inferiority of certain groups. In this scenario, those that are viewed as less equal have restricted access to basic services and treatments. It may result in policies which place restrictions on the rights and opportunities of those living with mental illness.

Despite decades of policy interventions to address stigma and enhance knowledge about mental illnesses, institutions remain stubbornly permeated by outdated and misleading beliefs.

The impact of stigma

People with mental health problems can experience discrimination (negative treatment) in all aspects of their lives. Stereotyping and prejudice can compound existing problems and result in poorer outcomes for individuals. The Mental Health Foundation (2022) report that nearly nine out of ten people with mental health issues

Figure 6.1: A stage model of self-stigma

Awareness and recognition of stereotype – 'I know what they think'

Agreement that the stereotype is valid – 'I think that they are right'

Application of stereotype to the self – 'I think they are right about me'

Harm – 'What's the point of trying, I'm not able'

Source: adapted from Corrigan and Rao (2012)

say stigma has had a negative impact on their lives. They note that people with a mental health condition are among the least likely of any group with a long-term health condition or a disability to:

- be in paid employment;
- be in a long-term relationship;

- secure high-quality accommodation;
- be socially included.

Some other harmful effects of stigma are:

- reluctance to seek help or treatment and to stay with treatment;
- social isolation;
- lack of understanding by family, friends, co-workers or others;
- fewer opportunities for work, school or social activities, or trouble finding housing;
- bullying, physical violence or harassment;
- health insurance that doesn't adequately cover mental illness treatment;
- the belief that you'll never succeed at certain challenges or that you can't improve your situation.

Table 6.1 shows that stereotypes and discrimination occur as a result of public, self- and institutional stigma.

Employment and stigma

Research has consistently indicated that most people with mental health problems want to be in paid employment (Drake and Wallach, 2020). Being in the workforce is associated with independence, self-esteem, self-confidence and social inclusion. Yet despite this willingness to work, people with mental health issues have much lower employment rates than the general population. While data on the specific role played by stigma is limited, it is clear that stigma is an important factor contributing to unemployment and underemployment, as across different countries and cultures, people with mental health issues face discrimination in the work setting. Stigma is a significant contributing factor to the disadvantaged labour market position of people with mental illness. This is a significant and complex issue and one that requires more research attention. Brouwers (2020) identifies four areas where stigma contributes to adverse employment outcomes for people with mental health problems:

Table 6.1: Stereotypes and discrimination in public, self- and institutional stigma

	Public stigma	**Self-stigma**	**Institutional stigma**
Stereotypes	People with mental illness are dangerous, incompetent, to blame for their disorder, unpredictable	I am dangerous, incompetent, to blame	Stereotypes are embodied in laws and institutional processes
Discrimination	Employers may not hire them, landlords may not rent to them, the healthcare system may offer them a lower standard of care	Lowered self-esteem and self-efficacy: 'Why try? Someone like me is not worthy of good health.'	Intended and unintended loss of opportunity

- Employers and other stakeholders in the employment context frequently hold negative attitudes towards people with mental health issues, and this decreases the chances of these people securing employment. Common beliefs are that workers will have low productivity levels and high rates of absence, they will need intensive supervision, and they will not be able to meet the demands of the workplace. Individuals with poor mental health are viewed as a homogenous group rather than individuals with varying needs and expectations. The stereotype that mental illness means an individual is dangerous or unpredictable is particularly damaging. Additionally, it is important that mental health support workers encourage and facilitate employment rather than depicting it as an unrealistic expectation. The danger is that this then becomes a self-fulfilling prophecy which increases the risk of long-term unemployment.
- Both disclosure and non-disclosure of mental health issues are problematic in the work environment. Due to fears about

discrimination or being labelled, workers hide mental health conditions from their peers and their managers. This is often accompanied by anxiety that disclosure of personal health conditions would not be kept in confidence and could become the subject of general workplace discussion. Expectations are that rather than being supported, individuals may find themselves ostracised or excluded. It is also feared that disclosing a condition would harm career progression and negatively impact opportunities. On the other hand, disclosure is critical to prevent poor outcomes such as stress, sickness or job loss. Occupational health can provide important forms of support and mitigation. Workplace managers are often trained in mental health issues and can provide bespoke support.

- Self-stigma limits job-seeking activities and prevents people from applying for employment opportunities. Anticipation of poor treatment and discrimination stops people from engaging in the job market or seeking promotion. The 'why try' phenomenon is a sense of futility that arises when people believe that they are not capable or not worthy of attaining personal goals. The application of stereotypes to oneself is associated with a diminished sense of self-worth.

- Stigma acts as a barrier to employment because it can prevent people with a mental illness from seeking available healthcare and support because of fear of being treated differently in the workplace. Even when support services are available, individuals are reluctant to seek help. Missing out on treatment presents a risk for worsening treatment, prolonged periods of sick leave and additional stress.

Language and stigma

Language is rarely neutral; rather, it is infused with meaning. The words we use shape how we see the world and ourselves. We have a choice in the words we use to describe ourselves, others and the world around us. The words we choose and the meanings we attach to them influence our decisions, beliefs and wellbeing.

In mental health, language is especially significant – the words we use shape how we view people with mental illness and our actions towards them. Language that conveys attitudes based on stigma encourages the viewing of stigmatised people with less regard and erodes their self-worth. Stigmatising language serves to maintain inequalities and reduce social justice. When used indiscriminately, words can create barriers, stereotypes and labels that are difficult to overcome. Labels can maintain hierarchical power differentials and reinforce disadvantage (Vojak, 2009). Certain ways of talking about mental illness can alienate members of the community, sensationalise the issue and contribute to stigma and discrimination. The use of language associated with mental health problems to describe everyday behaviours, and sometimes undesirable behaviours, trivialises and stigmatises the real-life experience of people living with a mental health disorder. Although mental health can be a tricky subject, that doesn't mean we should avoid discussing it. Language can empower individuals to discuss their issues and access support, thereby reducing harm. Table 6.2 shows some preferred language to use when communicating about mental illness.

Common misconceptions and myths about mental health

Although common misconceptions about mental illness may seem innocuous, they can be damaging in several ways. Mental health myths perpetuate toxic stereotypes that can keep people from getting the help they need. Some people may fear how others will view them if they come forward and ask for help. Others may avoid treatment because of misconceptions about the type of care they will receive. This can leave many people struggling on their own and internalising the negative views of mental illness, and this can ultimately make their problems worse. Some of the most common misconceptions are:

- All people with mental illnesses are crazy.
  Terms like 'crazy', 'nuts' and 'insane' are powerful words that feed into traditional stereotypes of mental illness. They perpetuate

Table 6.2: Language for communicating about mental illness

Dos	Don'ts	Why?
Do say the person is 'living with' or 'has a diagnosis of' mental illness	Don't say the person is a 'mental patient', a 'nutter', 'lunatic', 'psycho', 'schizo', 'deranged', 'mad'	Certain language sensationalises mental illness and reinforces stigma.
Do say the person is 'being treated for' or 'someone with' a mental illness	Don't say the person is a 'victim', 'suffering from', 'affected with' a mental illness	Some terminology suggests a lack of quality of life for people with mental illness.
Do say the person has a 'diagnosis of' or 'is being treated for' a mental illness	Don't say the person is 'a schizophrenic', 'an anorexic'	Labelling a person by their mental illness reinforces the idea they are different.
Do say the person's behaviour is 'unusual' or 'erratic'	Don't say the person is 'crazed', 'deranged', 'mad', 'psychotic'	Some descriptions of behaviour imply existence of mental illness and are inaccurate.
Do say 'antidepressants', 'psychiatrist' or 'psychologist', 'mental health hospital'	Don't say 'happy pills', 'shrink', 'mental institution'	Colloquialisms about treatment can undermine people's willingness to seek help.
Reword any sentence that uses psychiatric or media terminology incorrectly or out of context.	Don't say, for example, 'psychotic dog'. Don't use 'schizophrenic' to denote duality, as in 'schizophrenic economy'	Terminology used out of context adds to misunderstanding and trivialises mental illness.

Source: adapted from Everymind (2021)

the idea that mental illness is wild, uncontrollable and always severe when in fact there is a wide spectrum of mental illness and mental health disorders. They range from mild to more severe, and they may come and go. These terms are also often associated with symptoms like hallucinations and delusions, but these symptoms tend to be present only in specific mental health disorders.

- Mental illnesses and health disorders are extremely rare.

  Mental illnesses are so common that almost everyone will develop a psychological disorder at some stage in their life. For most people, this is temporary (Reuben and Schaefer, 2017). Most people will never receive treatment, but their lives may suffer. At any given time, approximately one quarter of the population is experiencing a mental illness. It is estimated that one in four people worldwide will experience poor mental health at some time (WHO, 2001). However, serious psychotic disorders like schizophrenia are estimated to occur in less than 1 per cent of the population and mental health disorders are often short-lived.

- Mental illnesses make people violent.

  One of the more common misconceptions about mental illness is that it makes people violent and dangerous. Schizophrenia and other psychotic disorders in particular have a reputation for violence. Yet people with poor mental health are more likely to be the victim of violent crime than the perpetrator.

- People with mental illness cannot function in society.

  Another of the more common myths associated with mental illness is that it makes the person unable to function in normal society. While some mental health disorders can be crippling, many people with mental illnesses are still productive members of society. Contrary to the stereotype, not all people with mental health disorders are locked away in secure units and separated from 'normal' society. Most people with mental health problems are employed and enjoy a family life.

- You cannot get better if you have a mental illness.

  It is a common misconception that once someone develops a mental illness, their life is changed forever. While some mental illnesses are chronic, treatment can help people learn how to better manage their symptoms and get more control over their disorder; in some cases, proper treatment can help people overcome their disorder almost completely. A substantial component of mental disorder is short-lived and of low severity. Many mental health disorders can be temporary and will not recur.

- Treatment is scary.

   Because of the images portrayed by the media, as well as the past use of controversial techniques, there are many misconceptions about mental illness treatment that can make people scared to get help. Shock therapy, straitjackets, padded rooms, lobotomies and a mess of pills that make the patient numb are mostly a thing of the past. Nowadays, treatment usually consists of a combination of therapy methods, like psychotherapy, and where necessary medication, which can be adjusted to avoid adverse reactions. Most people in residential facilities are there voluntarily.

Toxic masculinity

Both men and women are affected by poor mental health, but mental health issues among men are much more likely to go undiagnosed and untreated. Poor mental health, particularly among young men, can be viewed as a silent killer. Research suggests that sociocultural factors may partly explain this phenomenon. Masculine norms dictate acceptable behaviours and traits. In Western societies, men are subjected to a culture that may make expressing emotions such as distress or anxiety difficult (Milner et al, 2018; Chatmon, 2020). Patton et al (2018) note that differences in gender norms typically emerge in late childhood or early teens and quickly become entrenched.

Stigma often acts as a lens through which an individual's behaviour or characteristics are judged as socially acceptable. Toxic masculinity involves a set of expectations or guidelines stereotypically associated with the male gender role or manliness, which perpetuate ideas of strength, stoicism and power. Males should be strong, in control, competitive, not restricted by vulnerability (Rice et al, 2021). Men are believed to be transgressing their gender norms when they show signs of psychological distress or ask for psychological help. This is portrayed as a sign of weakness and vulnerability and can compromise norms about what being a man entails. There are multiple aspects of toxic masculinity, but there is broad agreement that it has three core components:

- Toughness – men should be physically strong, aggressive, dominant and self-reliant.
- Anti-femininity – men should not be associated with anything that is associated with showing emotion or requiring help.
- Power – men must have power and status to gain the respect of others. There is a need and desire to foster domination and control.

If a man violates an accepted male gender role, he may be marginalised and ostracised. He may be disqualified from full public acceptance if he appears feminine or weak. Diminished social status is the price for being perceived as 'unmanly'. Consequently, men may feel the need to adjust their behaviours or hide their distress to conform to expectations, regardless of the negative impact on their mental health. Toxic masculinity discourages men from seeking treatment for issues such as depression and loneliness, which are viewed as weaknesses. In this context, it is inappropriate for men to talk about their feelings and emotions.

Discouraging men from seeking help and promoting certain behaviours can have drastic consequences for individuals as well as society. Outdated ideas about what it means to be a man today, based on unrealistic cultural standards, can place unrealistic and unhealthy expectations on men and boys. Eliminating the stigma around mental illness is helped by encouraging men to ask for help and express their emotions. Men's poor mental health often goes undiagnosed and untreated, as they are less likely to seek help than women. Globally, depression and suicide are ranked as a leading cause of death among men. Masculine norms which outline acceptable behaviour are literally killing men. Phrases such as 'boys will be boys' or 'man up' reinforce ideas about accepted, appropriate behaviours.

Adherence to these rigid masculine norms may lead to:

- worsening of depression and anxiety;
- substance misuse;
- greater health risks (for cardiovascular and metabolic disease);
- issues with interpersonal intimacy;
- issues with domestic violence;
- aggression;
- increase in psychological distress;
- avoidance of help-seeking behaviours;
- homophobia.

There is increasing acceptance that the concept of a 'real man' is simply toxic masculinity – a damaging and outdated stereotype. This concept is perpetuated by society, encouraging men to repress emotions and feelings. Increasingly, there is acknowledgement that these ideas damage men and others in the process. Rice et al (2021) suggest that while gender norms are hard to shift, there is a need to promote a different kind of socialisation and emotional agenda. Engagement around the value systems of young males should avoid shaming their behaviours and focus on positive masculine traits so as to avoid the serious challenges to health that stem from restrictive gender norms.

Campaigns to address stigma

Given the far-reaching negative impacts of mental health stigma, this issue became a significant area of research in the 2000s, underpinned by substantial financial commitments from national governments and voluntary organisations. In response to increasing awareness of stigma and its consequences, a wide range of initiatives has been undertaken at national and international levels. Examples include the WHO's Closing the Gap, New Zealand's Like Minds Like Mine and Canada's

Opening Minds. Reviews of the evidence on programmes to reduce mental ill health stigma demonstrate that in some circumstances interpersonal contact and increased education can be an effective way of promoting positive attitudes (Henderson and Gronholm, 2018). Despite the increasing interest in anti-stigma interventions, there is considerable uncertainty about their impact. There is need for a greater understanding of what works and why. In the UK, there have been programmes to address stigma and discrimination in England, Scotland and Wales. Each of these anti-stigma interventions had a number of elements aimed at different target groups, such as young people and the media.

Large-scale projects are expensive and therefore it is crucial that they are fit for purpose. Globally, it is acknowledged that robust evaluation is critical to ensure that interventions are efficient and effective uses of resources. Due to the complex and complicated nature of stigma and the many obstacles to accessing care, any interventions for addressing this issue need to be tailored to local requirements. Population norms will impact on the validity, reliability and acceptability of initiatives. Evaluation of initiatives has highlighted the limited scope of interventions and confusing and poorly expressed objectives. Some anti-stigma campaigns have focused almost entirely on changing attitudes and stereotypes and challenging damaging ideas. Some have argued that this approach is too narrow and that it is not possible to address stigma without enhancing the social, economic and political rights of those living with mental illness (Sweeney and Taggart, 2018; Walsh and Foster, 2021). Reframing mental distress as a political issue facilitates a wider discussion about power and social inequality. Stigma can be viewed as a useful tool for those who wish to justify policies which exacerbate power imbalances. Rather than being depicted as an individual problem caused by insufficient resilience or weaknesses, stigma can be understood as a wider issue embedded in social and political systems.

Based on his review of stigma, Stuart (2016) highlights that in many countries, particularly low- and middle-income countries (LMICs), funding for mental health issues has been minimal and inadequate. As a result, many stigma reduction programmes have not been subjected to independent review or evaluation. While evidence in this field is increasing, it remains incommensurate with the burden associated with stigma. The cost-effectiveness of anti-stigma campaigns and their transferability remain subject to speculation. Identifying the key principles underpinning successful interventions should be prioritised. Poorly conceived anti-stigma programmes can have detrimental effects and rather than addressing social intolerance, have deepened it. Community-based programmes may set out with good intentions, but without a robust evidence base, they can flounder. Additionally, the anti-stigma advocacy community and the research community have different cultures of knowledge with different views of what constitutes 'evidence'. Reconciling the needs and wishes of these communities represents a significant challenge.

Stuart (2016) notes that advocacy groups for people with mental illness rarely have the funding, time or expertise to participate in in-depth monitoring, reflection and learning. Generally, formal evaluation programmes are beyond the financial means of these groups. Because they need knowledge that is contextualised, easily accessible, decision-oriented and pragmatic, they accept a much broader range of evidence and share it more informally. In this context, scientific knowledge – which is formal, objective and decontextualised, and has a lengthy peer-review process – is considered of lower value.

One of the world's longest-running anti-stigma campaigns, Time to Change, was launched in England in 2007 and ended in March 2021. It was England's most ambitious programme to address discrimination and stigma. This multifaceted campaign was based around a national marketing plan and community engagement involving service users, backed by celebrity endorsement. It encouraged employers to sign a pledge to support employees with mental health problems, raise awareness and reduce stigma in the workplace. It consisted of over 35 projects, including a nationwide awareness-raising campaign, a keep-fit project, roadshow events, social media engagement and local community projects. Prior to this, attempts in England to address poor mental health were fragmented and piecemeal. Overall findings for the project were mixed. On the one hand, it was associated with a modest change in public attitudes, but it is difficult to ascertain how much of this change was related specifically to the project. Between 2008 (the year before the campaign was launched) and 2011, there had been a significant fall in the level of discrimination experienced by people using mental health services in England and a small increase in the proportion of people who reported experiencing no discrimination (Corker et al, 2013). Early assessments concluded that the campaign was a low-cost and cost-effective intervention.

Anti-stigma campaigns play a role in reducing stigma and prejudice but should be part of a wider strategy to change attitudes and behaviours. Large, high-profile campaigns should be viewed as one component in a multidimensional approach. For instance, they could include efforts to address the impact of the media on stigma. There has been some improvement in this area. The tone and content of media articles covering mental health issues have improved over time. Research has noted a move away from negative stereotypes towards a more accurate and sympathetic portrayal of people with mental health problems (Chen and Lawrie, 2017) But while distorted images of mental illness are no longer commonplace in the media, many portrayals are still skewed towards negative stereotypes that sustain othering. Similarly, awareness-raising on its own can have limited results. The complex relationship between knowledge and prejudices was highlighted in a study by Chen and Lawrie (2017), which found that although knowledge of schizophrenia increased in a population sample between 2005 and 2017, perceptions of dangerousness and unpredictability did not. Raising awareness does not automatically lead to an improvement in the treatment of people who experience mental distress (National Survivor User Network, 2019).

To address the challenges presented by stigmatisation and othering of those impacted by mental health distress, it has been suggested that anti-stigma approaches may need to be informed by the complex interplay of factors that are often relevant. This would include recognition that mental illness may be a response to poverty, social exclusion and trauma. Framing mental health issues in this way can help to convey the relevance of social, political and economic factors. This positioning and reframing enables and encourages people to ask about power relations and why poor mental health is often linked to poverty and deprivation. A central question is: why has stigma remained so pervasive despite increased knowledge and national anti-stigma campaigns?

In dealing with power differentials and ensuring that campaigns and messaging are effective, it is crucial that projects and initiatives are led by people with lived experience of mental distress. Stigma disempowers and excludes people, perpetuating disadvantage and discrimination. But ensuring the voices of people who have been directly affected are front and centre of interventions can transform lives. To encourage help-seeking, services should embed trauma-informed approaches at all levels, thereby addressing power imbalances between providers and service users to ensure respectful practice. Conceptualising mental illness through survivor-led models with a focus on recovery should inform service design and delivery.

Time to Change Global was launched in 2018 in Ghana, Kenya, Nigeria, Uganda and India. The main aim of this project was to improve public attitudes and behaviour towards people with mental health difficulties in LMICs. Despite a growing body of evidence highlighting the prevalence of stigma in these countries, most interventions and research have been conducted in high-income countries. Time to Change Global was piloted using a series of social marketing campaigns, launched in Accra and Nairobi, alongside champions with lived experience of mental health issues, trained and supported by nongovernmental organisations to share their stories with local populations at 'social contact' events and then online during the COVID-19 pandemic.

Based on their review of anti-stigma campaigns, Walsh and Foster (2021) conclude that despite two decades of anti-stigma campaigns, people with mental illnesses continue to be othered. They note that evaluations of high-profile interventions show that these are weak and the concerns about their unintended consequences prevail. While there may be short-term attitude change, the evidence for sustained change in opinions is poor. The underlying conceptualisations of these initiatives are simplistic and fail to acknowledge the wide range of social processes that lead to 'them' and 'us' narratives. To date, there has been an absence of programmes designed to address the blame aspect of stigma. Also minimal attention has been paid to how the public makes sense of mental illness.

More recent assessments of anti-stigma campaigns have concluded that there is a considerable way to go in terms of promoting a nuanced understanding of how the public view mental illness (Hermaszewska et al, 2022). The early campaigns between 2000 and 2020 have been criticised for focusing on a largely biomedical explanation of mental illness, based on the medicalisation of human emotions and diagnostic labelling (Walsh and Foster, 2021). It has been suggested that the focus on the biomedical model of mental health encourages a 'them' and 'us' narrative rather than promoting the idea that mental health is a continuum; the latter has the ability to elicit a more positive public response (Thibodeau, 2020). To avoid the othering of individuals with mental disorders, people with lived experience have increasingly called for anti-stigma approaches that are informed by an understanding of mental distress as a response to social and economic exclusion, violence and human suffering (Sweeney and Taggart, 2018). Viewing mental distress through this lens facilitates a critical analysis of the relationship between power, mental health, stigma and discrimination. Using this framing can highlight psychosocial, medical and political dimensions. For example: whose knowledge and understanding of mental distress is being taught in stigma reduction efforts? Interventions should be informed by human rights approaches and survivor research.

Anti-stigma interventions for healthcare professionals

In recognition of the deleterious impacts of stigma, programmes to reduce stigma have been targeted at professionals who have high levels of contact with service users, those who are in a position of power and those who can improve outcomes. Stigma may be encountered in any walk of life, but in healthcare it is particularly egregious, negatively impacting people when they may be at their most vulnerable. Addressing the structural aspects of stigma that are embedded in the healthcare system has the potential to transform experiences for both providers and service users.

Interestingly, research has suggested many people with mental disorders report that contact with healthcare professionals is especially stigmatising (Thornicroft et al, 2006; Henderson et al, 2014; Knaak et al, 2017). Stigma related to mental illness pervades the healthcare sector. This has been described as a cultural issue, where staff in many healthcare settings are not comfortable dealing with mental rather than physical issues. They may display little empathy or understanding of recovery and may make certain people wait longer to be seen. Furthermore, mental health issues are viewed as more time-consuming and complex, negatively affecting the patient-provider relationship. There is a considerable body of evidence demonstrating that healthcare providers tend to hold pessimistic attitudes about the possibility and likelihood of recovery, which is experienced as a source of stigma and a barrier to recovery for people seeking help for mental illness (Knaak et al, 2017).

Often these professionals are dismissive of symptoms, appear sceptical and engage in labelling. People with mental health disorders often receive a lower quality of care for physical health issues, such as heart disease and diabetes, and this may be a contributing factor to lower life expectancy. Many report that their physical health issues are not taken seriously, and consequently they feel disempowered and marginalised. Health professionals exercise a considerable amount of power over service users, and it is therefore essential that they are fully trained on bias and discrimination. Professionals such as nurses and doctors can provide culturally appropriate anti-discriminatory healthcare that is cognisant of the complex effects of the social determinants of health. Stigma in healthcare undermines diagnosis, treatment and successful health outcomes. Addressing stigma is fundamental to delivering high-quality healthcare and achieving optimal results.

The following are key components of anti-stigma initiatives for healthcare providers:

- Incorporate social contact in the form of a personal testimony from a trained speaker with lived experience of mental illness.
- Use multiple forms or points of social contact – for example, a presentation from a live speaker and a video presentation, multiple first-voice speakers, multiple points of social contact between participants and people with lived experience of mental illness.
- Focus on behavioural change by teaching skills that help healthcare providers know what to say and what to do.
- Challenge stereotypes and unconscious bias.
- Ensure there is an enthusiastic facilitator or instructor who models a person-centred approach – a person-first perspective as opposed to a pathology-first perspective – to set the tone and guide programme messaging.
- Emphasise recovery.

Conclusion

Mental illness has a long history of stigmatisation across the world. Despite advances in knowledge and increased awareness, stigma persists. Stigma can lead to prejudice and discrimination that affects a person's ability to earn a living, access care and become a full member of society. Harmful stereotypes, such as depicting people with mental issues as dangerous or unpredictable, remain widespread. The consequences of stigma can be profound and devastating, hampering recovery and perpetuating mental distress.

It is not easy to shift attitudes and address stigma, but experience shows that change can happen. Knowledge is power, and stigma may be tackled through social contact and education. Research suggests that anti-stigma campaigns need to adopt both 'bottom up' and 'top-down' approaches.

Social contact interventions have been shown to be an effective way to reduce stigma. Education and training strategies targeted at healthcare professionals are a key component of anti-stigma campaigns. In order to address power imbalances and avoid othering, programmes should be led and co-designed by people with lived experience of mental distress.

Further reading

McKenzie, S.K., Oliffe, J.L., Black, A. and Collings, S. (2022) 'Men's experiences of mental illness stigma across the lifespan: a scoping review', *American Journal of Men's Health*, 16(1). doi: 10.1177/15579883221074789

Tyler, I. and Slater, T. (2018) 'Rethinking the sociology of stigma', *The Sociological Review*, 66(4): 721–43.

Vogel, D.L. and Wade, N.G. (eds) (2022) *The Cambridge Handbook of Stigma and Mental Health*, Cambridge: Cambridge University Press.

7

The media and mental health

Introduction

The media strongly influences expectations, norms and perceptions. For many people, the media is a key source of information about mental illness, and there is extensive evidence demonstrating how media coverage can influence public attitudes and perceptions of mental health. Movies and television shows, as well as other forms of entertainment, shape how people see the world. People often believe what they see and hear in the media, and this can trigger unhealthy thoughts and ideas. Social media has become an indispensable aspect of life in the modern world. The smartphone has become a constant companion, firmly embedded into everyday activities. The proliferation of online activities has sparked a debate about the pros and cons of social media. The main implications of this are twofold. First, social media can inform and educate on mental health issues. Online platforms have been used to disseminate positive messages and campaigns. However, the proliferation of misinformation about mental health is a growing concern. Online communities for mental health can expose individuals to false, damaging, misleading and dangerous information. Second, there is a growing body of work assessing the impact of the use of social media on mental health. Heavy use of social media is associated with depression, anxiety, poor sleep patterns and isolation (Karim et al, 2020; Meier, 2021; Azem et al, 2023).

Media stigmatisation of mental illness

It has been widely accepted that the media plays a key role in perpetuating stereotypes and negative public opinion about mental illness. Despite some progress in understanding of mental health, common stereotypes that those affected are unpredictable, dangerous, violent or incurable remain a staple in some sections of the media. Portrayal of exaggerated, inaccurate images of some psychiatric disorders for dramatic effect can result in the belief among the general population that people with a mental illness are best avoided. To a great extent, the media advises us who is to be praised and who is to be scorned. Even though only a very small minority of people with mental illness commit serious crimes or are associated with brutality, media representations tend to focus on violence and danger when portraying them. Research suggests that there is a hierarchy of mental health stigma. Schizophrenia and antisocial personality disorder were the most stigmatised diagnoses, and depression, generalised anxiety disorder and obsessive–compulsive disorder were the least stigmatised diagnoses (Hazell et al, 2022). Sensationalising and misrepresenting mental illness can be harmful to those living with serious mental health conditions. Also, importantly, this could discourage people who are suffering from speaking out. Those who are worried about their condition could feel shame and decide against seeking help, resulting in worse public health outcomes. Stigma is associated with avoidance of or delays in help-seeking, which can have profoundly negative consequences for the individuals involved. It is also strongly linked to non-adherence to treatment plans or withdrawal from services, which can result in adverse outcomes (Clement et al, 2015).

Nonfiction representations

When depicting mental illness, the media often resorts to overgeneralisation – for example, suggesting that every person with schizophrenia hallucinates, has delusions and appears disordered and unstable. In media reports, schizophrenia is associated with violence and erratic behaviour. The media has also exaggerated the association between schizophrenia and suicide. In her analysis of the portrayal of schizophrenia, Owen (2012) notes that the association with self-harm and suicide was inaccurate and misleading. Of particular concern is that the media portrays mental illness as a personal tragedy, something that is untreatable and unmanageable. Recovery is rarely the focus of films or television dramas.

Media portrayals of people with mental illness often skew toward either stigmatisation or trivialisation. Consequently, all forms of media – including television, films, magazines, newspapers and social media – have been criticised for disseminating negative stereotypes and inaccurate descriptions of people with mental illness. This poor representation across all forms of media has serious consequences and may turn real struggles with poor mental health into entertainment.

Media depictions of mental health problems are overwhelmingly focused on violence, and this appears to be a global trend (Pilgrim, 2017). Over three decades ago Hyler et al (1991) suggested that the 'homicidal maniac' was a particularly pejorative stereotype about people with mental illness. However, in recent years there have been some attempts to deal with mental health problems in a more empathic and nuanced manner. Modern media are beginning to rise to the challenge to give more serious consideration to mental illness, without resorting to tropes or cliches.

Research has consistently show that the news and entertainment media provide overwhelmingly negative and distorted images of mental illness, which emphasise force, unpredictability and dangerousness (see Stuart, 2016; Srivastava et al, 2018). People with poor mental health are depicted as inadequate or defective. There is also a tendency to stress negative reactions to people with poor mental health, including scorn, ridicule, rejection and social exclusion. The profound impact of this negative framing on people with mental health disorders is hard to overstate. It damages self-confidence, erodes trust and negatively affects help-seeking behaviours and adherence to treatment plans.

Fiction representations

The fictional portrayal of people with mental health problems in cinema and television is often misleading and stigmatising, and these depictions can have profound and lasting impact on public attitudes. This can reinforce stigmatisation in the real world. Byrne (2009) identified four main cinematic stereotypes of people with mental health problems: objects of fun and ridicule; fakers; people to be pitied; and people who are violent. Within the field of psychiatry, and indeed within broader medical contexts, it is widely accepted that the film *One Flew Over the Cuckoo's Nest* radically changed the public's perception of mental health and treatment, leading to high levels of mistrust and disgust in relation to treatment for mental illness (Domino, 1983). In this film, patients are brutally mistreated; they are portrayed as passive victims of an authoritarian inhumane regime. Its infamous horrifying portrayal of electroconvulsive therapy, with the patient's body wracked with high-voltage electricity as punishment, led to widespread revulsion at this treatment. Any potential therapeutic impact of this procedure was lost in the negative stereotyping.

Research for the Annenberg Inclusion Initiative assessed portrayals of mental health conditions in the 100 highest-grossing films at the US box office in 2016 and 2022 (Pieper et al, 2023). The findings paint a grim picture: mental health conditions were erased, dehumanised and stereotyped on screen. The portrayal of mental health was rarely authentic or nuanced. Less than 2 per cent of all speaking and named characters in both years were depicted with a mental health condition, and among the characters with a mental health problem, the majority were White, violent and disparaged by other characters. Content lacked depictions of help-seeking behaviours and did not highlight positive coping that ameliorated or reduced symptoms.

Portraying help-seeking behaviours in storytelling is one way to destigmatise mental health problems and even encourage viewers to consider available resources for their own needs. Unfortunately, as Pieper et al (2023) show, films failed to showcase positive actions to manage mental health conditions. Roughly a quarter of characters with mental health conditions were in therapy and a lower share was in treatment. The few characters who did engage in therapy or treatment were predominantly White and women, which obscures the reality that people from all backgrounds benefit from mental health interventions.

In 2019, the release of the film *Joker* caused controversy due to its depiction of severe mental illness. One of the more toxic ideas that the film subscribes to is that mental deterioration is associated with extremely violent behaviour. According to Driscoll and Husain (2019), mental health conditions such as psychosis remain shrouded in stigma and are poorly understood, and this representation of mental deterioration is irresponsible and a missed opportunity to explore wider social issues such as poverty and isolation. The lead character in *Joker*, Arthur, is a person with mental illness who becomes extremely violent. He has a complex mix of personality traits. The plot oscillates from a portrait of an individual who is struggling with mental disorder to a supervillain caricature (Skryabin, 2021). Scarf et al (2020) found that after viewing the film, people had higher levels of prejudice toward those with mental illness. Additionally, the authors suggest that '*Joker* may exacerbate self-stigma for those with a mental illness, leading to delays in help seeking.'

Pieper et al (2023) examined how characters with mental health conditions were portrayed across 300 films. The vast majority (almost 80 per cent) of characters with mental health conditions were subject to some type of denigration on screen. This could include general slurs that were not related to a character's mental health condition, almost half of characters (47 per cent) were disparaged specifically with respect to their mental health.

Mental health is rarely accurately portrayed in films. There are countless movies that use mental health illnesses and struggles in gimmicky and exploitative ways that are offensive, though sometimes even flawed movies can raise awareness about things many people are still reluctant to discuss. There are also movies that give eye-opening accounts at subjects not often dealt with in the mainstream.

The Netflix show *13 Reasons Why* has been trending around the world since its release in 2017. The show is about a girl named Hannah Baker, who tragically takes her life; she makes recordings beforehand in which she talks about the 13 reasons why she wants to die by suicide. The series deals with topics such as isolation and sexual assault while also romanticising suicide. It suggests to viewers that when a person dies by suicide, people pay more attention to their story. In this series, Hannah carefully plans and structures her death in a way that is very far from the reality of suicide. Most people who suffer from depression do not end their lives for attention; instead they are overcome with pain and complex emotions. It is particularly unrealistic to suggest that a teenager during an emotional crisis would have the time and ability to create a series of elaborate tapes. Unfortunately, the show doesn't educate viewers on the reality of suicide or how to get help; rather, it distorts suicide as a means of getting revenge.

The series has attracted a barrage of criticism for its depiction of depression and suicide. Mental health professionals have described the series as misleading and potentially triggering for vulnerable people at risk of suicide (Bernstein, 2019). In the show, depression and suicide are treated as high-school drama rather than serious mental health issues. Rosa et al (2019) have suggested the controversy around this popular show was largely due to the gap between intent and delivery of messages. It was intended to raise awareness of mental health problems and spark conversations about mental health and suicide. Instead, the show provides viewers with examples of self-harm and information on ways to self-harm. Rather than any exploration of distress or mental illness, suicide is depicted as the only solution. The way that it addresses suicidal ideation and prevention sustains rather than challenges stereotypes. Suicide is one of the leading causes of death for teenagers, and depression is a condition that afflicts millions of adolescents. Importantly, individuals of this demographic are especially susceptible to harmful media content. Consequently, understanding the link between mood, mental state, viewership and media content is critical for reducing the rate of adolescent suicide.

Media accounts tend to focus on the individual experience of mental illness rather than framing it as a societal issue. Consequently, those consuming media may perceive mental illness as the fault of the individual. Personality flaws or character weaknesses are believed to be the cause of problems. People with poor mental health are viewed as lazy or not trying hard enough. Individuals just need to 'pull themselves together' and 'snap out of it'. There is little consideration of the socioeconomic determinants of mental health, such as poverty, trauma or biological factors.

Social media

Given that social media platforms have radically changed the way we communicate with each other and how we access and digest information, there is an increasing focus on mental illness and the role of social media. On the one hand, inaccurate posts can lead to misleading ideas about the nature and development of poor mental health. On the other hand, sensitive, balanced, well-informed posts can challenge preconceptions, prejudices and stereotypes. Social media can be a powerful platform for mental health advocates and increase understanding of the experience of mental illness. Social media campaigns have the power to educate, inform and project positive news stories.

Oversimplification and trivialisation of mental illness

Within the media, some mental health disorders are oversimplified and the associated challenges minimised. Depression and anxiety are serious, often chronic, health conditions, which can become legally classified as disabilities. Equating depression with sadness or low mood exacerbates misunderstandings and dismisses the reality of living with serious illness. Anxiety and stress are not normal life challenges that can be overcome simply through mindfulness or breathing exercises.

The media can also trivialise mental illness by depicting it as less severe than it can be in reality. For example, obsessive-compulsive disorder (OCD) is a serious anxiety disorder where intrusive thoughts drive compulsive actions. It has been estimated that this illness affects 2.2 million Americans, with very different impacts (National Alliance on Mental Illness, 2012). Media portrayals of the condition tend to stereotype the compulsive aspect of the illness, such as repeated handwashing, checking of locks or organising of books. In addition, research has demonstrated that posts on social media platforms such as Twitter/X trivialise and mock OCD (Pavelko and Myrick, 2015). People with OCD are depicted as being overly concerned with perfection and cleanliness. The thoughts and processes that drive these behaviours are overlooked or ignored. This misrepresentation, suggesting OCD is a personality trait, is damaging for sufferers. The power and reach of this platform means the belittling of this debilitating condition has seeped into a large section of the public consciousness, negatively impacting general understanding of this disease. Comedic representations and mockery of OCD also add to the perception that it is not to be taken seriously. Mockery has been described as a type of humour which denigrates or maligns an individual or a group. It is also associated with bullying and can be used to reinforce assumed superiority (Pavelko and Myrick, 2015).

Often people with eating disorders such as anorexia nervosa feel that their condition is made out to be less severe than it really is. This is in part because portrayals in the media often minimise its seriousness and hide the severe consequences of the disease when in fact it has one of the highest mortality rates of any mental health condition. Up to 10 per cent of people with anorexia die within ten years of getting the disease and up to 20 per cent will die after 20 years (South Carolina Department of Mental Health, 2022). Rather than highlighting the dangers and struggles faced by those with poor mental health, posts on social media sites such as Instagram or TikTok glamourise the disorder and minimise the challenges of living with it. Some posts revere the conventional stereotype of young, White, fragile 'waif'.

Portrayal of gender and mental illness

An important misrepresentation in the media concerns gender stereotyping in relation to mental illness. Gender is correlated with the prevalence of certain mental disorders. Men are overrepresented in depictions of serious mental illnesses, such as psychoses, substance misuse, personality disorders and schizophrenia. Men are portrayed as violent and dangerous, while women are dependent, weak, incompetent, submissive and docile. Women are more likely to be associated with depression and clinical responses (Meyer et al, 2011). Through such portrayals, the media contributes to the construction and maintenance of gender stereotyping associated with mental illness. This social construction of gender roles is also apparent in the depiction of mental health professionals. Professionals are much more likely to be male than is the case in reality; also, male psychiatrists are likely to be depicted as lustful, strange social misfits, while female psychiatrists have been deprived of love and affection and are vengeful (Gabbard and Gabbard, 1992). Female psychiatrists are often portrayed as acting unprofessionally and transgressing ethical boundaries of the client-patient relationship.

Portrayal of suicide and self-harm

Suicide is a global health issue. The WHO (2023) estimate that it is the fourth leading cause of death among 15- to 29-year-olds. Despite the relatively high prevalence, until relatively recently in the UK suicide was a taboo subject. For centuries, suicide was viewed a heinous sin, and it was hidden and associated with shame and guilt. This meant that people who were feeling suicidal didn't feel free to discuss their thoughts, fearing they would be viewed as a burden. Friends and family members are often unsure if they should ask someone if they are feeling suicidal. Self-harm is also poorly understood and usually associated with suicidal thoughts. Self-harm is a pattern of repetitive and non-suicidal behaviour, but it does increase the risk of suicide in the future.

Depictions of suicide in the media can have both detrimental and beneficial effects on suicidal behaviour. Discussing and describing suicidal behaviour can be thought of as treading a fine line between informing and promoting. Traditional and emerging media depictions of suicide have been identified as a key factor in influencing an individual's decision to attempt to take their own life. The impact of media reporting on this subject is complex and there are ongoing attempts to regulate it. Research into death by suicide has identified a copycat phenomenon termed the 'Werther effect' (Phillips, 1974; Ha and Yang, 2021). This refers to the fact that media reporting of suicides by well-known figures both in real life and fiction leads to a spike in suicides in the general population. Such reports could have a triggering effect, leading to copycat behaviours and increased levels of self-harm. Content that promotes suicide and self-harm can take various forms, including images and videos sharing tips, memorial pages that romanticise and glamourise suicide, and online challenges that encourage people to take part in harmful behaviours.

Conversely, research (Niederkrotenthaler et al, 2010) has highlighted the 'Papageno effect', where stories of individuals overcoming a suicidal crisis can reduce suicidal behaviour. Responsible social media posts can have a profoundly positive impact and can even save lives. One of the most powerful benefits online platforms can achieve is to raise awareness of an important issue and direct people to appropriate support. The stigma associated with poor mental health means many are reluctant to discuss their concerns with friends and family. Some support organisations, such as the Samaritans and Lifeline, use social media sites to provide access to up-to-date reliable resources. Others provide online counselling, discussion forums and safe spaces in which to talk and get professional help. For people living in rural or remote locations, social media can help address barriers to support, including lack of transport links.

The rise of social media platforms such as Twitter/X, Facebook and Instagram has renewed interest in the effect of media on suicides. To date, it is unclear if social media platforms are simply usurping the role of print media in reporting high-profile suicides or if the interactive aspect of social media plays a role in shaping responses. However, suicide is a significant public issue and it is neither realistic nor appropriate to suggest that it should not be discussed (WHO, 2023). The reaction to the death of actor Robin Williams shocked the world. His death led to a spike in the number of suicides, but there was also a marked increase in the number of suicide helplines and an increase in referrals to mental health support (Fink et al, 2018). His tragic passing illustrated the complex nature of reporting and discussing suicide. The growth of social media and online resources has radically transformed the way suicide and self-harm are presented and accessed by consumers, particularly younger users. The explosion in the use of smartphones globally means individuals, particularly young people, are more exposed to adverse and dangerous mental health messaging. The internet can be an invaluable source of support for young people who are struggling to cope with mental health issues. It can inform, educate and signpost users to help and support. The ability to communicate with peers who have experienced similar issues can help dispel myths and address misinformation. The growth of digital media has huge potential to deliver positive outcomes in mental health, particularly in the area of suicide prevention. Social media can be a powerful tool to educate and raise awareness about mental health and wellbeing, and it can help to normalise help-seeking behaviours and offer a range of support to those who may not otherwise have access to it.

Cyberbullying of children and young people

Bullying is not a new phenomenon, but developments in the digital landscape have fundamentally altered the way people experience it. As technology advances, so too do opportunities to connect with people across the world. However, unfettered communication is not always a positive thing, particularly for young people. Cyberbullying is online harassment. It includes any form of antisocial behaviour that uses technology, such as stalking, trolling, grooming and other online abuse designed to cause distress. For young people who may already be struggling to deal with the challenges of adolescence, cyberbullying can have catastrophic effects on their mental health. There is no universally accepted definition of cyberbullying, which hampers attempts to protect victims via legislation and the criminal justice system. According to Hinduja and Patchin (2014, p 11), it is purposeful and recurrent harm directed through digital devices platforms, such as computers and smartphones. Online bullies and stalkers frequently pursue their victims under fake online profiles. Cyberbullying, or electronic aggression, has already been designated a serious public health threat (Ferrara et al, 2018; Maurya et al, 2022).

While cyberbullying has been portrayed as a rising epidemic among children and adolescents, research has found that it rarely happens in isolation (Wolke et al, 2017). There are various settings where this behaviour takes place, including online forums and chat rooms. Wilful and repeated victimisation occurs using computers, social media and computer games. For example, Twitter/X is a hotbed of dangerous trolling that can leave long-lasting emotional scars. Examples of cyberbullying include:

- spreading malicious and damaging rumours;
- sending threatening or intimidating texts and emails;
- repeated and targeted harassment via social media;
- posting personal details online;
- using gaming sites to bully;
- blackmail and threats to expose embarrassing behaviour;
- posting inappropriate content without consent;
- fraud, theft or deception;
- stalking and continually commenting negatively;
- grooming.

Cyberbullying can affect a child's psychological wellbeing and academic performance, particularly when the bullying is linked to the child's school life. It does not stop at the end of the school day, but can continue at all hours of the day or night. The 24/7 nature of social media means that there is no escaping from the harassment or humiliation. Victims of this type of toxic behaviour can be bombarded relentlessly with messages, images and videos. In this context, there are no teachers to intervene to put a halt to it. Children who are the victims often try to hide these experiences from their parents and other adults. Peers who witness these behaviours are frightened to intervene in case they become targets too. This silence enables the toxic culture to continue unchecked.

Multiple studies have demonstrated that young people who are cyberbullied are at an increased risk of a number of mental health issues, including low self-esteem, loneliness and depression (Van Geel et al, 2014; Palermiti et al, 2017). Significantly, victims of cyberbullying among adolescents are at an increased risk of future mental health problems even if the level of victimisation is low (Fahy et al, 2016). Children may resort to negative coping mechanisms, such as drug and alcohol consumption, self-harm and suicide ideation. Intervention should be informed by traditional approaches to bullying, because the root cause of the harassment is likely to be similar.

There is extensive evidence demonstrating that the COVID-19 pandemic negatively impacted young people's mental health due to social isolation and loneliness during lockdowns and prolonged school closures. The loss of routine was particularly challenging for schoolchildren and may have a long-term detrimental impact on their mental health (El-Osta et al, 2021).

Safe and responsible media coverage

Numerous resources and guidelines for responsible media reporting have been published. The WHO (2000) has published a range of resources for professionals working in the field of mental health. The Samaritans have also produced a media guide on reporting suicide, which sets out guidance for documentaries, drama and news reporting (Samaritans, nd).

The media has a huge influence on norms, perceptions and attitudes: it has the ability to shape how we understand a wide range of issues. Misleading or poorly framed depictions of mental health can negatively impact people who are dealing with mental illnesses. Sensationalising tragic events or reporting intricate details of suicides should be avoided. It is essential that those engaged in reporting are fully cognisant of the adverse consequences of insensitive or inappropriate reporting. Generalisations based on hearsay and sensationalised expressions such as 'epidemic of suicide' or 'tsunami of suicide' or 'suicide capital of the world' should be avoided.

Before publishing stories, journalists and editors should consider the potential effects on families and other survivors in terms of stigma and psychological suffering. Sensational reporting in explicit detail of suicides or self-harm, especially if a celebrity is involved, may be considered legitimate news, but can be extremely dangerous. Detailed descriptions of the method used and how items were procured should be completely avoided.

In print media, news of a death should not appear on the front page with a banner or large font headline that mentions suicide. The method of suicide (for example, 'jumped from a building') should not be included in the headline. Mentioning the full name or other personal information of the deceased or attempter, or printing a photograph or location, may give a wrong signal to vulnerable people, suggesting that suicide can make them famous. The reason for suicide must not be oversimplified. Suicide never occurs due to a single factor or event but is the result of a complex interaction of several factors, and often the person has a background of psychosocial problems. It should be emphasised that while the overt cause of the suicide was the precipitating event, this was not the only cause. While publicising specific aspects of the person's background that may have played a causative role is neither necessary nor desirable, the presence of prior issues should be acknowledged. Any history of psychiatric disorders or drug misuse should be mentioned. A range of factors including mental illness and adverse life events can increase the risk of suicide.

In television news reports, suicide cases should not be presented as the headline story unless they involve public interest. Repetitive and excessive reporting of the events should be avoided. Glorification of suicide victims as martyrs may encourage vulnerable persons to imitate the behaviour to attract media attention. Highlighting the adverse consequences of deliberate self-harm (brain damage, paralysis and so on) may deter future attempts.

Impact of social media on mental health

There can be little doubt that the proliferation of social media has a significant impact on the mental health of users, but within the literature there is intense debate about its benefits and risks (Boer et al, 2020; Valkenburg, 2022; Zsila and Reyes, 2023).

Research in 2022 reported that people spent 2.3 hours daily on social media (Braghieri et al, 2022; Faulhaber et al, 2023). However, it is the manner of use that determines whether use is harmful or beneficial factor. The effects of social media on mental health are complex, as different goals are served by different behaviours and different outcomes are produced by distinct patterns of use.

There is evidence to suggest that those who limit their time on social media are likely to be happier than those who do not (Faulhaber, et al 2023). Prolonged use of social media sites may be linked to negative manifestations and symptoms of depression, anxiety and stress (O'Reilly et al, 2018; Vahedi and Zannella, 2021). In their extensive study of mood disorders, Lyall et al (2018) found that those who logged onto Facebook before bedtime were 6 per cent more likely to have a major depressive disorder and rated their happiness level 9 per cent lower than those with better sleep hygiene. Research by Thai et al (2023) found that young people were spending, on average, six to eight hours per day on screens, most of this on social media.

Platforms such as YouTube, TikTok, Instagram, and Snapchat are increasingly popular, particularly among younger people. Individuals use social media for many reasons, including shopping, gaming, dating and networking, as well as to boost self-esteem, promote health and gain access to critical medical information. Connections made through social media can enhance a sense of community and belonging. They provide opportunities to engage with people with similar interests. Social media platforms may provide invaluable forums to explore concerns and address challenges. They can offer peer support, encourage help-seeking behaviours and allay fears and anxieties (Naslund et al, 2020). For those who are socially isolated and feel marginalised, online communities provide ways of sharing experiences and obtaining emotional and practical support. This can boost self-esteem and encourage a sense of belonging.

Given the shortfalls in the quality, availability and reach of mental health services across the UK, these platforms may provide alternative opportunities to secure support. The anonymity afforded by social media offers a safe space for people to express themselves and reveal their personal experiences with mental illness. In other words, they allow self-expression without the danger of stigma. Self-disclosure can be an important therapeutic element and is linked to psychological and physical wellbeing; individuals may choose to withhold their identities, allowing themselves more candid disclosure than may be possible offline (Suler, 2004). Social media platforms are ideally placed to signpost those experiencing mental health issues to organisations that can provide help and support. They can also connect to others who have experienced issues themselves and motivate people who are vulnerable to seek help.

Social media can provide important motivational tools for those who want to achieve a range of healthy lifestyle goals, such as quitting smoking, losing weight, reducing alcohol intake or joining a gym. Publicising an intent to achieve a goal on social media promotes accountability to others and can create a support network. It can also encourage others to get involved – a classic example of social contagion. Some research suggests that sharing a goal publicly not only promotes accountability but helps one stay focused, dramatically increasing the chances of success though research specifically on the effect of sharing goals on social media is limited.

Conversely, it can be argued that social media has fractured society, with the race for shares of 'likes' and 'followers' creating a toxic culture that is detrimental to mental health. Social media networks have become an inherent part of modern culture, but they are addictive and can be toxic. The algorithms used by sites direct service users to the most extreme posts and videos to boost engagement and revenue. Young people are increasingly living their lives online, and this comes with a number of serious risks. Unrealistic expectations and distorted views of reality can have a negative impact on mental health. The constant stream of uncensored, unregulated messages and posts has serious downsides. The culture of comparison is one of the most significant difficulties with social media. Platforms such as Instagram depict idealised versions of people's lives – perfect houses, perfect bodies and perfect holidays – creating unrealistic standards. The airbrushing and filtering of reality creates distorted views of life. The illusion that others are living a perfect lifestyle can create feelings of unhappiness and envy. The quest for perfection can have a profound impact on emotional wellbeing and is associated with heightened levels of anxiety and depression among social media users, particularly young people (Miller et al, 2024). The constant need for validation through posting perfect images online can create a sense of relentless pressure.

Heavy social media usage has been linked to anxiety, loneliness and depression (Dhir et al, 2018; Reer et al, 2019), which can aggravate mental health problems. Several studies have likened the symptoms of excessive social media use to addiction. It produces a surge of dopamine in the brain, and this keeps people coming back for more. This 'high' from social media use becomes more and more difficult to resist. Likes and reposts provide instant gratification, leading to compulsive behaviours. Patterns of addictive behaviour are associated with compromised decision-making, decreased sleep quality, depression, anxiety and stress (Meshi, 2019; Hussain and Wegmann, 2021).

Body image

An important debate around the use of social media relates to its impact on body image and how this affects mental health. Given the growing use of social media, it is likely to have a significant impact on body image issues, both positive and negative. On the one hand, it can provide access to a range of support systems, advice and information about health and fitness. Inspirational content can motivate and challenge people to address issues around self-confidence due to poor body image. On the other hand, extensive social media use potentially can have harmful effects.

To date, it has been the negative impacts on self-esteem that have attracted attention. Extensive exposure to representations of the ideal body image may cause dissatisfaction and despair, and it may be a predictor of poor mental health and eating disorders (Prnjak et al, 2021). The internalisation of unattainable beauty ideals leads to greater levels of dissatisfaction with body shape and appearance. Regular comparison with others can exacerbate insecurities. Thai et al (2023) found that vulnerable teenagers and young adults who reduced their social media by 50 per cent for a few weeks reported a significant improvement in their self-esteem. While anyone might feel that they don't quite measure up to the ideal, for vulnerable individuals with eating disorders or body image disorders, such as body dysmorphic disorder, representations of the ideal body may be particularly detrimental. Body dysmorphic disorder is associated with a preoccupation with a slight or non-existent flaw in appearance. Compulsive and time-consuming behaviours, such as constant checking for problems and seeking reassurance, can be substantially worsened by social media.

Pro-anorexia, also known as pro-ana, websites project a positive depiction of anorexia nervosa and other eating disorders. Thinness is correlated with perfection, love, happiness and success. Rather than acknowledging that people with anorexia are suffering from a recognised illness, they are lauded for showing restraint and self-control in relation to food. These online communities may reinforce misinformation and promote dangerous, risky behaviours and messages. For example, these sites promote harmful behaviours by stressing thinness, restriction and compensatory activities.

In some instances, online content may be considered life-threatening. Individuals are encouraged to hide their disorder from friends and family and not to access treatment and support. Pro-ana can also correlate with self-harm or suicide, as many people who believe in the pro-ana message glamourise other forms of emotional distress too. It is well established that the media plays a key role in promoting beauty ideals and norms, but the link between social media and eating disorders is a particular cause for concern. Social media platforms are different from traditional print and broadcast media, as they offer interactivity and access to a community of like-minded individuals (Perloff, 2014). Social media platforms such as Instagram, TikTok, Snapchat and YouTube make it easy to share pro-ana content with millions of people instantaneously. Users can share restrictive diet plans, 'thinspirational' images and toxic quotes about starvation or thinness, and they can edit their photos in order to share a distorted goal (Aparicio-Martinez et al, 2019). Exposure to this type of content is associated with reduced self-confidence and increased dissatisfaction with body image.

With regard to mental health, the explosion in the use of social media in the last decade can be thought of as a double-edged sword. Studies have highlighted the benefits of platforms in terms of allowing people to express their feelings and access support. However, other research (Zubair et al, 2023) has highlighted the link between excessive social media use and psychological problems. This relationship is not, though, straightforward, as there are a range of contributory factors. For example, the impact on adolescents may be different to the impact on older people, and the time spent online and the type of content consumed will affect outcomes.

FOMO

FOMO (fear of missing out) is a relatively new term to describe a phenomenon observed on social networking sites. In 2015, it was included in the Oxford English Dictionary. FOMO includes two processes: perception of missing out followed with a compulsive behaviour to maintain social connections (Gupta and Sharma, 2021). FOMO is associated with a range of negative perceptions and linked to poor sleep patterns, anxiety, negative self-perception and inability to deal with rejection. There is a body of evidence assessing the links between FOMO and poor mental health (Elhai et al 2020; Luca et al, 2020). This work concludes that FOMO undermines good mental health and interferes with quality of life. Liu et al (2023) contend that effective interventions to reduce negative impacts need to assess what type of social interactions are sought by individuals. They found that positive solitude did not affect mental health, but FOMO was linked to detrimental effects. Also strengthening social connections can help individuals deal with feelings of disconnectedness and provide opportunities for interactions.

Conclusion

The media plays a crucial role in shaping perceptions of mental health conditions. However, despite advances in knowledge and understanding, the portrayal of mental illness has changed relatively little over time. Characters with mental illness are often associated with danger, unpredictability and a lack of hope. Films continue to perpetuate the link between mental health and violence. Outdated stereotypes have a negative impact on attitudes and beliefs of audience members. However, when mental health experiences are depicted in a nuanced, empathic manner, this can decrease stigma and promote help-seeking behaviours.

Social media has become an indispensable feature of modern life. While social media platforms have revolutionised the way we communicate and share information, it is essential to acknowledge the potential negative consequences they may have on mental health when used excessively or irresponsibly. Undoubtedly, these platforms have provided multiple benefits and opportunities for individuals worldwide, but they have also raised concerns regarding their potential negative effects on mental health. Unrelenting exposure to comparison with the seemingly perfect lives of others, cyberbullying and excessive screen time are examples of how social media can contribute to mental health issues such as low self-esteem, depression and anxiety. A better understanding of the impact of social media is essential to enable us to recognise problems, set boundaries and monitor use of online platforms. The digital world poses particular challenges and presents opportunities in terms of mental health. It is important that we recognise and acknowledge both the positive and negative aspects of this method of communication.

Further reading

House, A. and Brennan, C. (2023) *Social Media and Mental Health*, Cambridge: Cambridge University Press.

Valkenburg, P.M., Meier, A. and Beyens, I. (2022) 'Social media use and its impact on adolescent mental health: an umbrella review of the evidence', *Current Opinion in Psychology*, 44: 58–68.

Conclusion

Globally, poor mental health is a critical and growing public health challenge, with significant inequalities existing both within and between countries. There is increasing recognition that enhancing the mental health of the population should be moved up the public policy agenda. For too long, mental health has been the Cinderella service in terms of the lack of funding and the low level of policy attention it attracts. Chronic underfunding and lack of suitably qualified staff have a major impact on the quantity and quality of care available. When it comes to the resourcing and scope of care, there is still an unacceptable divergence in the way we treat physical illness and mental illness.

There has been much change in the long history of mental healthcare. From 1247 until the 1700s, Bethlem Hospital in London was the only mental asylum in the UK. By the 1700s, there were a few private institutions where wealthy people with mentally ill relatives could have them incarcerated. Treatments were cruel and many patients did not survive. Most of what happened in mental asylums was based on a lack of knowledge and a belief that mental ill health is a disease of the body rather than the mind. In the mid-1700s, medical and social reformers began to agitate for change, and at the beginning of the 1800s, social reformers spearheaded a change in attitudes that led to local authorities providing purpose-built accommodation for mentally ill patients.

By the mid-19th century, public asylums had adopted a new model of non-restraint for patients. This required larger numbers of staff who were better trained to operate the new model of care and was a major change in emphasis from 'custody to cure'. Despite this, in the early 1900s, mental hospitals were overcrowded, underfunded and, while offering better care, were more about control rather than cure.

Treatments were still based on the assumption that mental illness has a physical cause, and they continued to be cruel and experimental, without evidence of success. Mental illness remained stigmatised and was thought of as incurable.

When the NHS was established in the UK in 1948, funding was concentrated in physical healthcare. In 1962, the NHS Hospital Plan for England and Wales proposed a programme of hospital building and the closure of asylums, mainly driven by an awareness of human rights. It was not until 1971 that a government paper (Killaspey, 2006) proposed abolishing asylums and delivering services in general hospitals or integrating former patients into the community with the support of GPs and social services. This included supported housing, day care centres and community-based mental health nurses and social workers. The National Health Service and Community Care Act 1990 passed responsibility for what had become known as care in the community to local authorities. As no extra funding was allocated to carry out this extra responsibility, services were inadequate and unevenly provided. This, along with repeated reform of health services and the establishment of NHS trusts, added to what Scull (2021) describes as 'chaos'.

Care in the community was controversial. Media reports of several high-profile murders carried out by psychiatric patients created a 'moral panic', causing policy and legislation to be informed by public safety and risk management. The Mental Health Act 1983 (amended in 2007) for England and Wales has been undergoing reform, with a Draft Mental Health Bill proposed in 2022, after it was found that a disproportionate number of Black and minority ethnic groups are being detained under the Act. There are also proposals for a reduction in the use of the Act for detention of people with a learning disability or autism. The draft legislation to reform the Mental Health Act proposes to make it fit for purpose in the 21st century.

While deinstitutionalisation has been a long and slow process, community care represents a major policy shift in mental health services. However, critics have pointed to a lack of adequate planning and a resulting burden on families, and parity of esteem between physical and mental health services continues to be an aspiration.

Nonetheless, with community-based mental health services, multidisciplinary mental health teams, modern therapies, greater public awareness and some progress in reducing stigma, there is now better understanding of the importance of mental health and wellbeing.

Of course, much work is required to reverse the decades of neglect in mental health services. Across the world, governments have not devoted sufficient energy and resources to address the needs of people with mental illness. While we have come a long way in the last few decades, there remains a long way to go before mental health is fully understood as an area of policy and practice.

The book emphasises that our understanding of the causes of mental health have moved beyond a medicalised understanding focused largely on the brain. There is no consistent biological evidence to suggest that all mental health disorders are due to dysfunction in the brain. Many common mental health disorders, such as depression and anxiety, are related to psychological and environmental factors. The history of psychiatry can be characterised by a shifting focus from biological to social explanations of mental health. The broad acceptance of the biopsychosocial model reflects the recognition that biological, psychological and social factors shape mental health and illness.

Another key issue highlighted in the book is that mental health issues are not distributed equally across the population, and people who are socially disadvantaged have a much greater risk of poor mental health. Poor mental health is among the most prevalent and disabling health conditions across the globe. Although many disorders have biological roots, they are also substantially influenced by modifiable social, economic and environmental conditions that affect individuals, communities and populations. Various aspects of these environments affect mental wellbeing at different stages of life. In the UK, a gulf of almost two decades has emerged in the life expectancy of people with and without some forms of mental illness (WHO, 2022c). In one of the richest countries of the world, this huge differential is a damning indictment of care given and care not given. The relationship between low income and mental illness is complex – causality can run in both directions – but the gap between the rich and the poor in terms of the likelihood of experiencing mental illness remains huge. This was compounded by the COVID-19 pandemic, as this affected poor people's mental health most (Banks and Xu, 2020; BMJ, 2021). Those on the lowest incomes paid the highest price in terms of mental health. Within the literature on mental health, there is increasing support for taking a life course approach to tackle the social determinants of mental health. Alongside this, there is a wealth of evidence to support a focus on early intervention and prevention. It is also crucial to think about long-term policies that build strong communities and empower the people who live in them. The link between social determinants and mental disorders is thought to be partially related to the accumulation of stress, although this can be mitigated by building resilience and providing a range of support. A healthy community can be a critical component of good mental health. Being part of a community can create a sense of belonging and foster a sense of positivity, and social interaction can prevent loneliness and isolation. Strategies to enhance social cohesion can help to make people feel empowered and reduce the risk of poor mental health.

To address people in impoverished communities being at a heightened risk of mental illnesses, economic disparities and societal-level issues need to be addressed through cross-governmental public policy interventions. The social determinants of mental health can be viewed through the lens of social justice and mitigated through advocacy, political will and risk-based policy interventions. Yet, despite research demonstrating the cost-effectiveness of early intervention to prevent and treat common mental disorders, delivery at scale and translation into real-world benefits has been slow.

Despite mental health problems affecting an estimated one in four people globally (WHO, 2001, 2022c), stigma remains very powerful and is a significant societal problem. The pernicious effects of stigma may represent the single greatest barrier to the development of mental health programmes worldwide, affecting political support, charitable fundraising and the priority afforded to support for national and local services. Institutional stigma extends to research and clinical practice, from the low status of psychiatry as a clinical and academic specialty to the meagre portion of research spending on mental health relative to its disease burden.

Among the public, knowledge of mental health problems is poor and negative beliefs and attitudes are widespread. Both are key elements of stigma. One of the most common and damaging misperceptions is that people with schizophrenia are violent and a danger to others. This view has been perpetuated by misleading media reports and portrayals that focus largely on negative information and rely on tired tropes about mental illness. The preoccupation with danger simply serves to reinforce the stigma associated with emotional distress. The culture of individual blame and the use of negative language when discussing mental illness further serves to marginalise and exclude. People with mental illness internalise stereotypes, leading to guilt and shame. The explosion in social media has largely been depicted as having negative implications for mental health. For example, hashtags during the COVID-19 pandemic promoted ageism and generated intergenerational conflict. On the other hand, social media sites such as Facebook, Instagram, Twitter/X and TikTok are now recognised as important platforms for educating, informing and challenging misconceptions.

The insidious effects of stigma, including from discrimination and prejudice, have increasingly been recognised by governments and policy makers as an area where action is needed. Despite increased awareness, stigma continues to persist throughout the world, perpetuating barriers to seeking care. We know that the severity of public stigma varies depending on the nature of the mental illness – for instance, schizophrenia and substance use disorders are associated with higher levels of stigma. Recently, a number of 'anti-stigma' initiatives have been implemented to promote equality for people with mental illness. The extent to which these have led to change in attitudes and behaviours is debated within the literature. There is a growing consensus that programmes that are based solely on changing attitudes are inadequate given the scale of the challenge; instead, a range of approaches are needed to tackle stigma. Reducing stigma can dramatically improve the quality of life of those with a mental health problem and should be a major priority.

Worldwide, there are difficulties in obtaining valid, reliable data on levels of mental ill health. Many countries do not delineate their healthcare spending budgets and mental health is integrated into wider health budgets. What data is available points to chronic underfunding in mental health services for adults and children. This has led to long waiting lists and inadequate resourcing and staffing levels, which applies also to the diverse offering of community-based mental health services.

The economic case for investing in the prevention of mental health conditions has been well established. Many mental health problems are preventable, and it is counterproductive to wait until problems arise before providing support. There is a wealth of evidence demonstrating the cost-effectiveness of programmes that can prevent poor mental health. The vast majority of mental illnesses start before the age of 18, but the services available for children and young people remain woefully inadequate. It is impossible to ignore the human and financial costs of not providing appropriate care.

By focusing on the prevention of poor mental health, we can reduce both economic and personal costs and support more people to live mentally healthy lives. Rather than waiting for people to become unwell and seek treatment, governments and decision makers should commit to policies that promote good mental health and invest in community programmes that empower everyone, especially people at higher risk, to live well. Training people and giving them the skills and techniques to manage their own wellbeing is essential.

Work by organisations such as the Mental Health Foundation demonstrates the success of initiatives such as parenting programmes, anti-bullying programmes and workplace support. Not only are people supported to have good mental health, but there are significant cost savings. For example, Bonin (2011) found that for every £1 spent on parenting programmes, £9.30 could be saved in the long term through reduced costs in the health, education and criminal justice sectors.

The WHO (2022c) *World Mental Health Report* highlights that community mental healthcare is consistently underfunded. It would be feasible to assume this refers to low-income countries, and it probably does. However, this is also the position in the UK. The worst example of the lack of parity between physical and mental healthcare concerns the emergency mental healthcare available in the event of a mental health crisis, which is described as suicidal behaviour, panic attacks, severe anxiety, psychosis and being out of control. It has been found that people experiencing a mental health crisis do not know where to go for support, and there are no clear referral routes and no single point of access (Care Quality Commission, 2015; Royal College of Psychiatrists, Scotland, 2021). In 2021, NHS England estimated that there were eight million people with mental health needs who were not in contact with mental health services (National Audit Report, 2023).

Investment is being made in England to address need, with 24/7 NHS helplines, mental health teams being rolled out in schools and colleges for early intervention and capital investment in crisis response and emergency care. The Community Mental Health Framework for Adults and Older Adults (NHS England, 2019b) has replaced the Care Programme Approach for adults with serious mental illness, which had been in effect for around three decades. It is intended to provide a personalised approach based on an assessment.

As access to services has been an issue, some public services in the UK are adopting the 'no wrong door' approach. The Royal College of Psychiatrists in Scotland called on the 2021–26 Scottish Parliament to use this approach in addressing mental health needs in Scotland, noting that the existing system was confusing, disjointed and creates delays to accessing treatment. Their members have reported patients having to go through multiple channels to be seen and facing delays, finding their appointment is not with the right professional or service and going back to the bottom of the waiting list, and having to travel miles to be seen.

The voluntary, community and social enterprise (VCSE) sector is a valuable partner in the provision of mental health services. Some VCSE organisations provide services in the local community, and there are also national organisations that lobby for changes to policy. Partnership with the VCSE sector has become a priority for government. VCSE organisations can be more accessible than statutory services – for example, they have been found to suit the needs of young men by providing drop-in services with instant access and peer support (Betts and Thompson, 2017). However, VCSE organisations can depend on the government and statutory services for funding, which is short term and leads to uncertainty and loss of knowledge when staff have to move on due to lack of funding for their post. Austerity has meant they have been asked to do more for less money, and procurement methods can mean a small organisation will spend several weeks filling in a tender that ultimately may be unsuccessful, or have to train its staff in the General Data Protection Regulation or safeguarding even though this is not included in the funding allocation. Integrated health and social care in England is being delivered across England by 42 integrated care systems. They allocate the NHS budget and commission local services. They are required to work with local organisations to address the health needs in their area.

Since the introduction of the National Health Service and Community Care Act 1990, UK legislation has made it a requirement to involve service users in planning services. User groups offering mutual support and charitable organisations lobbying for better mental health services had been growing since the 1970s, and by 2005 there were around 500 groups involving carers and service users wanting more involvement in decisions about support. Co-production of services and person-centred care are now familiar in healthcare policy, although co-production is not clearly defined and can mean different things to different people, groups and organisations.

The concept of recovery from mental illness emerged alongside the deinstitutionalisation in the 1970s. Lobbying by service user groups led to mental health services adopting recovery as one of the overall aims of care (Roberts and Boardman, 2013). Implementing Recovery through Organisational Change (ImROC) was a three-year project (2009–12) involving the NHS, the VCSE sector and service users and carers in 29 sites in England. The ImROC project led to the establishment of recovery colleges throughout the UK. These provide an example of co-production in action. They are embedded in the community and are committed to recovery. People recovering from mental illness are supported through education, with courses co-designed by those with learned experience of mental illness and tutors. Recovery colleges offer different courses depending on the priorities of those involved in their design. They work with provider partnerships or host organisations. Reviews suggest (Perkins et al, 2018) that they benefit service users and staff and demonstrate attainment of recovery goals. However, their estimated budget represents less than 1 per cent of NHS mental health spending (Research Into Recovery, nd).

The services offered by the VCSE sector and the recovery colleges provide care in the community near to a person's home – this is an aim that has been stated in policies of successive governments. They also represent value for money and are popular with service users, offering person-centred care, social interaction and community involvement.

Mental illness remains a complex and contested area. While significant progress has been made, particularly in addressing attitudes towards mental illness and the development of services, it can also be argued that the main barrier to the development of effective and sustainable mental health promotion strategies and initiatives has been, and continues to be, the contested nature of the concept of mental health.

Glossary

A&E	Accident and Emergency
ADHD	attention deficit hyperactivity disorder
APA	American Psychological Association
BDD	body dysmorphic disorder
CAMHS	Child and Adolescent Mental Health Services
CBT	cognitive behavioural therapy
CPA	Care Programme Approach
CTO	community treatment order
DoLS	Deprivation of Liberty Safeguards
DSM	Diagnostic and Statistical Manual of Mental Disorders
ECT	electroconvulsive therapy
FOMO	fear of missing out
GABA	gamma-aminobutyric acid
GP	general practitioner
IAPT	Improving Access to Psychological Therapies
ICD	International Classification of Diseases
ICS	integrated care system
ImROC	Implementing Recovery through Organisational Change
LGBTQ+	lesbian, gay, bisexual, transgender and queer (or questioning)+
LMIC	low- and middle-income country
MAOI	monoamine oxidase inhibitor
MDT	multidisciplinary team
NDRI	norepinephrine-dopamine reuptake inhibitor
NHS	National Health Service
NICCY	Northern Ireland Commissioner for Children and Young People

NICE	National Institute for Health and Care Excellence
OCD	obsessive-compulsive disorder
OECD	Organisation for Economic Co-operation and Development
PTSD	post-traumatic stress disorder
SCIE	Social Care Institute for Excellence
SEND	special educational needs and disabilities
SNRI	serotonin and noradrenaline reuptake inhibitor
SSRI	selective serotonin reuptake inhibitor
UK	United Kingdom
VCSE	voluntary, community and social enterprise
WHO	World Health Organization
YLD	year lived with disabilities

References

Abril, E.P., Tyson, K. and Morefield, K. (2022) 'SnapChat this, Instagram that: the interplay of motives and privacy affordances in college students' sharing of food porn', *Telematics and Informatics*, 74: 101889. doi: 10.1016/j.tele.2022.101889

Adler, N.E. and Rehkopf, D.H. (2008) 'US disparities in health: descriptions, causes, and mechanisms', *Annual Review of Public Health*, 29: 235–52.

Albert, P.R. (2015) 'Why is depression more prevalent in women?', *Journal of Psychiatry and Neuroscience*, 40(4): 219–21.

Allen, J., Balfour, R., Bell, R. et al (2014) 'Social determinants of mental health', *International Review of Psychiatry*, 26(4): 392–407.

All Party Parliamentary Group on Mental Health (2015) *Parity in Progress? The All Party Parliamentary Group on Mental Health's Inquiry into Parity of Esteem for Mental Health* [Online], Available: www.mind.org.uk/media-a/4405/appg-parity-in-progress-final.pdf (Accessed 13 July 2024).

Alonso, J., Liu, Z., Evans-Lacko, S. et al (2018) 'Treatment gap for anxiety disorders is global: results of the World Mental Health Surveys in 21 countries', *Depression and Anxiety*, 35(3): 195–208.

AM v SLAM NHS Foundation Trust (2013) UKUT 365 (AAC), [2013] MHLO 80 [Online], Available: www.mentalhealthlaw.co.uk/AM_v_SLAM_NHS_Foundation_Trust_(2013)_UKUT_365_(AAC),_(2013)_MHLO_80 (Accessed 20 March 2024).

Anon (1998) 'View point', *Mental Health Today*, July/August, p 37.

Anthony, W.A. (1993) 'Recovery from mental illness: the guiding vision of the mental health service system in the 1990s', *Psychological Rehabilitation Journal*, 16(4): 11–23.

APA (American Psychiatric Association) (2018) *DSM-5 Update*, APA Publishing.

APA (American Psychiatric Association) (nd-a) 'What are impulse control and conduct disorders?' [Online], Available: www.psychia try.org/patients-families/disruptive-impulse-control-and-cond uct-disorders/what-are-disruptive-impulse-control-and-conduct (Accessed 23 November 2023).

APA (American Psychiatric Association) (nd-b) 'What is psychotherapy?' [Online], Available: www.psychiatry.org/patients-families/psychotherapy (Accessed 14 March 2023).

Aparicio-Martinez, P., Perea-Moreno A.J., Martinez-Jimenez, M.P. et al (2019) 'Social media, thin-ideal, body dissatisfaction and disordered eating attitudes: an exploratory analysis', *International Journal of Environmental Research and Public Health*, 16(21): 4177. doi: 10.3390/ijerph16214177

Arias, D. Saxena, S. and Verguet, S. (2022) 'Quantifying the global burden of mental disorders and their economic value', *eClinicalMedicine*, 54(101675).

Arnstein, S. (1969) 'A ladder of community participation', *Journal of the American Institute of Planners*, 35(4): 216–24.

Asher, L. and De Silva, M.J. (2017) 'A little could go a long way: financing for mental healthcare in low and middle-income countries', *Epidemiology and Psychiatric Sciences*, 26(3): 248–51.

Avison, W.R. (1992) *Risk Factors for Children's Conduct Problems and Delinquency: The Significance of Family Milieu,* Paper presented at the American Society of Criminology Annual Meeting, New Orleans.

Azem, L., Al Alwani, R., Lucas, A. et al (2023) 'Social media use and depression in adolescents: a scoping review', *Behavioral Science*, 13(6): 475. doi: 10.3390/bs13060475

Baker, C. and Gheera, M. (2020) 'Mental health: achieving "parity of esteem"', *House of Commons Library* [Online], 16 January, Available: https://commonslibrary.parliament.uk/mental-health-achieving-parity-of-esteem/ (Accessed 10 June 2023).

Baker, C. and Kirk-Wade, E. (2024) *Mental Health Statistics: Prevalence, Services and Funding in England*, House of Commons Library [Online], Available: https://commonslibrary.parliament.uk/resea rch-briefings/sn06988/ (Accessed 20 March 2024).

Baldessarini, R.J., Tondo, L., Pinna, M. et al (2019) 'Suicidal risk factors in major affective disorders', *British Journal of Psychiatry*, 215(4): 621–6. doi: 10.1192/bjp.2019.167

Balogun, B. and Garratt, K. (2022) *Suicide Prevention: Policy and Practice*, House of Commons Library [Online], 25 January, Available: www.careknowledge.com/media/52501/cbp-8221.pdf (Accessed 24 March 2024).

Bamford Centre for Mental Health and Wellbeing (2011) *Troubled Consequences: A Report on the Mental Health Impact of the Civil Conflict in Northern Ireland*, Belfast: Commission for Victims and Survivors.

Banks, J. and Xu, X. (2020) 'The mental health effects of the first two months of lockdown and social distancing during the Covid-19 pandemic in the UK', Institute for Fiscal Studies.

Barclay, S. (2023) 'Government action on major conditions and diseases, statement made on 24 January 2023' [Online] Available: https://questions-statements.parliament.uk/written-sta tements/detail/2023-01-24/hcws514 (Accessed 20 March 2024).

Barros, P., Ng Fat, L., Garcia, L. et al (2019) 'Social consequences and mental health outcomes of living in high-rise residential buildings and the influence of planning, urban design and architectural decisions: a systematic review', *Cities*, 93: 263–72.

Baxter, L. and Fancourt, D. (2020) 'What are the barriers to, and enablers of, working with people with lived experience of mental illness amongst community and voluntary sector organisations? A qualitative study', *PLoS ONE*, 15(7): e0235334. doi 10.1371/ journal.pone.0235334

BBC News (2022) 'Muckamore Abbey Hospital: bad practices "allowed to persist"' [Online], 6 June, Available: www.bbc.co.uk/ news/uk-northern-ireland-61685339 (Accessed 30 March 2023).

Bekalu, M.A., McCloud, R.F. and Viswanath, K. (2019) 'Association of social media use with social well-being, positive mental health, and self-rated health: disentangling routine use from emotional connection to use', *Health Education & Behavior*, 46(suppl 2): 69S–80S.

Bell, A. and Allwood, L. (2019) *Arm in Arm: The Relationships between Statutory and Voluntary Sector Mental Health Organisations*, London: Centre for Mental Health.

Bell, A. and Pollard, A. (2022) *No Wrong Door: A Vision for Mental Health, Learning Disabilities and Autism Services in 2032*, London: NHS Confederation and Centre for Mental Health.

Bell, R., Donkin, A. and Marmot, M. (2013) *Tackling Structural and Social Issues to Reduce Inequities in Children's Outcomes in Low to Middle-Income Countries*, Office of Research Discussion Paper 2013-02, Florence: UNICEF Office of Research.

Beresford, P. (2019) '"MAD" Mad studies and advancing inclusive resistance', *Disability & Society*, 35(8): 1337–42.

Beresford, P. and Rose, D. (2023) 'Decolonising global mental health: the role of mad studies', *Cambridge Prisms: Global Mental Health*, 10: e30. doi: 10.1017/gmh.2023.21

Beresford, P., Nettle, M. and Perring, R. (2010) *Towards a Social Model of Madness and Distress?* York: Joseph Rowntree Foundation.

Bergmark, M., Bejerholm, U. and Markstrom, U. (2017) 'Policy changes in community mental health: interventions and strategies used in Sweden over 20 YEARS', *Social Policy and Administration*, 51(1): 95–113.

Bernard, M. (2017) 'Psychoanalysis versus psychotherapy: what's the difference?', *Mental Health Digest* [Online], 14 August, Available: http://insidefamilycounseling.com/psychoanalysis-versus-psychotherapy-whats-the-difference/ (Accessed 14 March 2023).

Bernstein, A. (2019) '13 reasons why: what the controversial drama gets wrong', *The Guardian*, 30 August, Available: https://www.theguardian.com/tv-and-radio/2019/aug/30/13-reasons-why-netflix-liberty-high#:~:text=Rather%20than%20give%20an%20honest,commitment%20to%20kindness%20and%20friendship (Accessed 6 September 2024).

Bester, K.L., McGlade, A. and Darragh, E. (2022) 'Is co-production working well in recovery colleges? Emergent themes from a systematic narrative review', *The Journal of Mental Health Training, Education and Practice*, 17(1): 48–60.

Betts, J. and Thompson, J. (2017) *Mental Health in Northern Ireland: Overview, Strategies, Policies, Care Pathways, CAMHS and Barriers to Accessing Services*, Research and Information Service Paper [Online], 24 January, Available: www.niassembly.gov.uk/globalassets/documents/raise/publications/2016-2021/2017/health/0817.pdf (Accessed 23 March 2024).

Beyari, H. (2023) 'The relationship between social media and the increase in mental health problems', *International Journal Environmental Research Public Health*, 20(3): 2383. doi: 10.3390/ijerph20032383.

BMJ (2021) Editorial 'Poverty, health and Covid 19'. *BMJ* 2021; 372: n376.

Boer, M., Van Den Eijnden, R.J., Boniel-Nissim, M. et al (2020) 'Adolescents' intense and problematic social media use and their well-being in 29 countries', *Journal of Adolescent Health*, 66(6), S89–S99.

Bogic, M., Njoku, A. and Priebe, S. (2015) 'Long-term mental health of war-refugees: a systematic literature review', *BMC International Health and Human Rights*, 15: 29. doi: 10.1186/s12914-015-0064-9.

Bonin, E.M., Stevens, M., Beecham, J. et al (2011) 'Costs and longer-term savings of parenting programmes for the prevention of persistent conduct disorder: a modelling study', *BMC Public Health*, 11: 803. doi: 10.1186/1471-2458-11-803

Bouras, N., Ikkos, G. and Craig, T. (2018) 'From community to meta-community mental health care', *International Journal of Environmental Research and Public Health*, 15(4): 806. doi: 10.3390/ijerph15040806

Bourke, J. (2021) 'Historical perspectives on mental health and psychiatry', in G. Ikkos and N. Bouras (eds) *Mind, State and Society: Social History of Psychiatry and Mental Health in Britain 1960–2010*, Cambridge: Cambridge University Press, pp 3–12.

Boyle, D. and Harris, M. (2009) *The Challenge of Co-Production: How equal partnerships between professionals and the public are crucial to improving public services*, NEF and NESTA.

Braghieri, L., Levy, R. and Makarin, A. (2022) 'Social Media and Mental Health', SSRN doi.org/10.2139/ssrn.3919760

Bratti, M., Mendola, M. and Miranda, A. (2015) *Hard to Forget: The Long-Lasting Impact of War on Mental Health*, IZA Discussion Paper No 9269, Bonn: IZA.

Brouwers, E.P.M. (2020) 'Social stigma is an underestimated contributing factor to unemployment in people with mental illness or mental health issues: position paper and future directions', *BMC Psychology*, 8, 36. doi: 10.1186/s40359-020-00399-0

Brown, G.W. and Harris, T. (1978) *The Social Origins of Depression*, London: Tavistock Press.

Bunting, B.P., Murphy, S.D., O'Neill, S. et al (2012) 'Lifetime prevalence of mental health disorders and delay in treatment following initial onset: evidence from the Northern Ireland Study of Health and Stress', *Psychological Medicine*, 42(8): 1727–39.

Byrne, P. (2009) *Screening Madness: A Century of Negative Movie Stereotypes of Mental Illness*, London: Time to Change.

Campbell, D.E. (2009) 'Civic engagement and education: an empirical test of the sorting model', *American Journal of Political Science*, 53(4): 771–86.

Campo-Arias, A. and De Mendieta, C.T. (2021) 'Social determinants of mental health and the Covid-19 pandemic in low-income and middle-income countries', *The Lancet Global Health*, 9(8): E1029–E1030.

Care Quality Commission (2015) 'Right Here, Right Now. People's experiences of help, care and support during a mental health crisis', [Online]. Available: www.cqc.org.uk/sites/default/files/20150630_righthere_mhcrisiscare_full.pdf (Accessed: 22 November 2024).

Carpenter, J., Schneider, J., Brandon, T. et al (2003) 'Working in multidisciplinary community mental health teams: the impact on social workers and health professionals of integrated mental health care', *British Journal of Social Work*, 33(8): 1081–103.

Castrodale, M.A. (2015) 'Mad matters: a critical reader in Canadian mad studies', *Scandinavian Journal of Disability Research*, 17(3): 284–6.

CDC (Centers for Disease Control and Prevention) (2022) 'Adverse Childhood Experiences (ACEs)'. [Online]. Available at: https://www.cdc.gov/violenceprevention/aces/about.html

Centre on Society and Health (2015) 'Why education matters to health: exploring the causes', *Virginia Commonwealth University* [Online], 13 February, Available: https://societyhealth.vcu.edu/work/the-projects/why-education-matters-to-health-exploring-the-causes.html#gsc.tab=0 (Accessed 23 March 2024).

Chang, E.S., Kannoth, S., Levy, S. et al (2020) 'Global reach of ageism on older persons' health: a systematic review', *PLOS ONE*, 15(1): e0220857. doi: 10.1371/journal.pone.0220857

Charlson, F., van Ommeren, M., Flaxman, A. et al (2019) 'New WHO prevalence estimates of mental disorders in conflict settings: a systematic review and meta-analysis', *The Lancet*, 394(10194): 240–8.

Chatmon, B. (2020) 'Males and mental health stigma', *American Journal of Men's Heath*, 14(4): 1557988320949322. doi: 10.1177/1557988320949322

Chen, M. and Lawrie, S. (2017) 'Newspaper depictions of mental and physical health', *British Journal Psychology Bulletin*, 41: 308–13.

Chien, W.T., Leung, S.F., Yeung, F.K. et al (2013) 'Current approaches to treatments for schizophrenia spectrum disorders, part II: psychosocial interventions and patient-focused perspectives in psychiatric care', *Neuropsychiatric Disease and Treatment*, 9: 1463–81.

Clark, D.M. (2019) 'IAPT at 10: achievements and challenges', *NHS England* [Blog], 13 February, Available: www.england.nhs.uk/blog/iapt-at-10-achievements-and-challenges/ (Accessed 14 March 2023).

Clement, S., Schauman, O., Graham, T. et al 'What is the impact of mental health-related stigma on help-seeking? A systematic review of quantitative and qualitative studies', *Psychological Medicine*, 45(1): 11–27.

Coalition for Personalised Care (2022) *Developing our Understanding of the Difference Co-Production Makes in Social Care*, London: SCIE.

Cohen, P. and Cohen, J. (1984) 'The clinician's illusion', *Archives of General Psychiatry*, 41(12): 1178–82.

Cole-King, A. and O'Neill, S. (2018) 'Suicide prevention identification, intervention and mitigation of risk', in L. Gask et al (eds) *Primary Care Mental Health* (2nd edn), Cambridge: Cambridge University Press, pp 103–24.

Compton, M.T. and Shim R.S. (2015) 'The social determinants of mental health', *Focus:* The Journal of Learning in Psychiatry, 13(4): 419–25.

Connolly, J., Munro, M., Macgillivray, S. et al (2022) 'The leadership of co-production in health and social care integration in Scotland: a qualitative study', *Journal of Social Policy*, 52(3): 620–39.

Cooper, D. (1967) *Psychiatry and Anti-Psychiatry*, London: Routledge.

Corcoran, P., Griffin, E., Arensman, E. et al (2015) 'Impact of the economic recession and subsequent austerity on suicide and self-harm in Ireland: an interrupted time series analysis', *International Journal of Epidemiology*, 44(3): 969–77.

Corker, E., Hamilton, S., Henderson, C. et al (2013) 'Experiences of discrimination among people using mental health services in England 2008–2011', *British Journal of Psychiatry*, 202(suppl 55): s58–s63.

Corrigan, P. (2004) 'Target-specific stigma change: a strategy for impacting mental illness stigma', *Psychiatric Rehabilitation Journal*, 28(2): 113–21.

Corrigan, P. (2008) 'Understanding and influencing the stigma of mental illness', *Journal of Psychosocial Nursing and Mental Health Services*, 46(1): 42–8.

Corrigan, P. (2018) *The Stigma Effect: Unintended Consequences of Mental Health Campaigns*, New York: Columbia University Press.

Corrigan, P. and Shapiro, J.R. (2010) 'Measuring the impact of programs that challenge the public stigma of mental illness', *Clinical Psychology Review*, 30(8): 907–22.

Corrigan, P. and Rao, D. (2012) 'On the self-stigma of mental illness: stages, disclosure, and strategies for change', *Canadian Journal of Psychiatry*, 57(2): 464–9.

Corrigan, P.W. and Bink, A.B. (2016) 'The stigma of mental illness', *Encyclopaedia of Mental Health*, 4(1): 230–4.

Corrigan, P. and Watson, A. (2002) 'Understanding the impact of stigma on people with mental illness', *World Psychiatry*, 1(1): 16–20.

Corrigan, P., Larson, J.E. and Rusch, N. (2009) 'Self-stigma and the why try effect: impact on life goals and evidence-based practices', *World Psychiatry*, 8(2): 75–81.

Corrigan, P.W., Rafacz, J. and Rüsch, N. (2011) 'Examining a progressive model of self-stigma and its impact on people with serious mental illness', *Psychiatry Research*, 189(3): 339–43.

Corrigan, P.W., Bink, A.B., Schmidt, A. et al (2016) 'What is the impact of self-stigma? Loss of self-respect and the "why try" effect', *Journal of Mental Health*, 25(1): 10–5.

Cummins, I. (2018) 'The impact of austerity on mental health service provision: a UK perspective', *International Journal of Environmental Research and Public Health*, 15(6): 1145. doi: 10.3390/ijerph15061145

Department of Health (1975) White Paper 'Better Services for the Mentally Ill', HMSO.

Department of Health (2012) *Preventing Suicide in England: A Cross-Government Outcomes Strategy to Save Lives* [Online], Available: https://assets.publishing.service.gov.uk/government/uploads/system/uploads/attachment_data/file/1183518/Preventing-Suicide-in-England-withdrawn.pdf (Accessed 19 July 2024).

Department of Health (2015) *Mental Health Act 1983: Code of Practice* [Online], Available: www.gov.uk/government/publications/code-of-practice-mental-health-act-1983 (Accessed 20 July 2024).

Department of Health and Social Care (2015) *Building the Right Support: A National Plan to Develop Community Services and Close Inpatient Facilities for People with a Learning Disability and/or Autism Who Display Behaviour that Challenges, Including Those with a Mental Health Condition* [Online], Available: www.england.nhs.uk/learning-disabilities/natplan/#:~:text=The%20national%20plan%20–%20Building%20the,and%20close%20some%20inpatient%20facilities (Accessed 20 July 2024).

Department of Health and Social Care (2017) *Five Year Forward View for Mental Health*. The Mental Health Taskforce, Available: https://www.england.nhs.uk/wp-content/uploads/2016/02/Mental-Health-Taskforce-FYFV-final.pdf (Accessed 6 September 2024).

Department of Health and Social Care (2018) *Modernising the Mental Health Act: Increasing Choice, Reducing Compulsion. Final Report of the Independent Review of the Mental Health Act 1983* [Online], Available: www.gov.uk/government/publications/modernising-the-mental-health-act-final-report-from-the-independent-review (Accessed 20 July 2024).

Department of Health and Social Care (2022) 'Better mental health support for people in crisis'. [Online], Available at: https://www.gov.uk/government/news/better-mental-health-support-for-people-in-crisis (Accessed 7 August 2024).

Department of Health and Social Care (2023) 'Major conditions strategy: case for change and our strategic framework', Updated August 2023. [Online], Available at: https://www.gov.uk/governm ent/publications/major-conditions-strategy-case-for-change-and-our-strategic-framework/major-conditions-strategy-case-for-cha nge-and-our-strategic-framework--2 (Accessed 8 August 2024).

Department of Health (Northern Ireland) (2018) *Co-Production Guide for Northern Ireland: Connecting and Realising Value through People* [Online], Available: www.health-ni.gov.uk/publications/co-pro duction-guide-northern-ireland-connecting-and-realising-value-through-people (Accessed 11 July 2024).

Department of Health (Northern Ireland) (2019) *Protect Life 2: A Strategy for Preventing Suicide and Self Harm in Northern Ireland 2019-2024* [Online], Available: www.health-ni.gov.uk/protectlife2 (Accessed 3 June 2023).

Department of Health (Northern Ireland) (2021) *Mental Health Strategy 2021–2031* [Online], Available: www.health-ni.gov.uk/ sites/default/files/publications/health/doh-mhs-strategy-2021-2031.pdf (Accessed 20 March 2024).

Department of Health (Northern Ireland) (2023) *Protect Life 2: A Strategy for Preventing Suicide and Self Harm in Northern Ireland 2019–2024. Progress Report* [Online], Available: https://.health-ni.gov. uk/sites/default/files/publications/health/doh-protect-life-2-act ion-plan-march-2023.pdf (Accessed 3 June 2023).

Department of Health (Northern Ireland) (nd) 'Bamford Review of Mental Health and Learning Disability' [Online], Available: www. health-ni.gov.uk/articles/bamford-review-mental-health-and-learn ing-disability (Accessed 9 March 2023).

Department of Health, Social Services and Public Safety (2006) *Protect Life: a Shared Vision – Suicide Prevention Strategy for Northern Ireland*, Belfast: DHSSPS.

Department of Health, Social Services and Public Safety (2010) *Review of the Evidence Base for Protect Life – A Shared Vision: The Northern Ireland Suicide Prevention Strategy Final Report*, National Suicide Research Foundation and DHSSPS.

Department of Health, Social Services and Public Safety (Northern Ireland) (2012a) *Child and Adolescent Mental Health Services: A Service Model* [Online], Available: www.health-ni.gov.uk/publications/child-and-adolescent-mental-health-services-service-model-july-2012 (Accessed 11 July 2024).

Department of Health, Social Services and Public Safety (2012b) *The Northern Ireland Suicide Prevention Strategy (Refreshed) 2012–2014*, Belfast: DHSSPS.

Dhir, A., Yossatorn, Y., Kaur, P. et al (2018) 'Online social and media fatigue and psychological wellbeing—a study of compulsive use, fear of missing out, fatigue, anxiety and depression', *International Journal of Information Management*, 40: 141–52.

Diamond, B., Parkin, G., Morris, K. et al (2003) 'User involvement: substance or spin', *Journal of Mental Health*, 12(6): 613–26.

Domino, G. (1983) 'Impact of the film, "One Flew Over the Cuckoo's Nest," on attitudes towards mental illness', *Psychological Reports*, 53(1): 179–82.

Drake, R.E. and Wallach, M.A. (2020) 'Employment is a critical mental health intervention', *Epidemiology and Psychiatric Sciences*, 29, e178 1–3.

Drake, R.E. and Whitley, R. (2014) 'Recovery and severe mental illness: description and analysis', *Canadian Journal of Psychiatry*, 59(5): 236–42.

Driscoll, A. and Husain, M. (2019) 'Why *Joker*'s depiction of mental illness is dangerously misinformed', *The Guardian* [Online], 21 October, Available: https://.theguardian.com/film/2019/oct/21/joker-mental-illness-joaquin-phoenix-dangerous-misinformed (Accessed 25 March 2023).

Duncan, F., Baskin, C., McGrath, M. et al (2021) 'Community interventions for improving adult mental health: mapping local policy and practice in England', *BMC Public Health*, 21(1): 1691. doi: 10.1186/s12889-021-11741-5

Education and Training Inspectorate (2018) *An Evaluation of the Effectiveness of Emotional Health and Well-Being Support for Pupils in Schools and EOTAS Centres* [Online], Available: www.etini.gov.uk/ sites/etini.gov.uk/files/publications/evaluation-of-emotional-hea lth-and-well-being-support-in-schools-and-eotas_0.pdf (Accessed 14 March 2024).

Eghigian, G. (2014) 'The First World War and the legacy of shellshock', *Psychiatric Times*, 31(4), [Online], Available: www. psychiatrictimes.com/view/first-world-war-and-legacy-shellshock (Accessed 20 July 2024).

Elhai, J.D., Gallinari, E.F., Rozgonjuk, D. et al (2020) 'Depression, anxiety and fear of missing out as correlates of social, non-social and problematic smartphone use', *Addictive Behaviors*, 105: 106335. doi: 10.1016/j.addbeh.2020.106335

Ellison, M.L., Belanger, L.K., Niles, B.L. et al (2018) 'Explication and definition of mental health recovery: a systematic review', *Administration and Policy in Mental Health and Mental Health Services Research*, 45(1): 91–102.

El-Osta, A., Alaa, A. and Webber, I. (2021) 'How is the COVID-19 lockdown impacting the mental health of parents of school-age children in the UK? A cross-sectional online survey', *British Medical Journal* Open, 11(5): e043397. doi: 10.1136/bmjopen-2020-043397

Erriu, M., Cimino, S. and Cerniglia, L. (2020) 'The role of family relationships in eating disorders in adolescents: a narrative review', *Behaviour Sciences*, 10(4): 71. doi: 10.3390/bs10040071

Ettman, C.K., Abdalla, S.M., Cohen, G.H. et al (2020) 'Prevalence of depression symptoms in US adults before and during the Covid-19 pandemic', *JAMA Network Open*, 3(9): e2019686. doi:10.1001/ jamanetworkopen.2020.19686

Fahy, A.E., Stansfeld, S.A. and Smuk, M. (2016) 'Longitudinal associations between cyberbullying involvement and adolescent mental health', *Journal of Adolescent Health*, 59(5): 502–9.

Farbstein, D., Lukito, S., Yorke, I. et al (2022) 'Risk and protective factors for self-harm and suicide in children and adolescents: a systematic review and meta-analysis protocol', *BMJ Open*, 12(11): e058297. doi: 10.1136/ bmjopen-2021-058297

Farina, A. (1998) 'Stigma', in K.T. Mueser and N. Tarrier (eds) *Handbook of Social Functioning in Schizophrenia*, Needham Heights, MA: Allyn & Bacon.

Faulhaber, M.E., Lee, J.E. and Gentile, D.A. (2023) 'The effect of self-monitoring limited social media use on psychological well-being', *Technology, Mind, and Behavior*, 4(2): doi: 10.1037/tmb0000111

Fell, B. and Hewstone, M. (2015) *Psychological Perspectives on Poverty*, London: Joseph Rowntree Foundation.

Ferrara, P., Ianniello, F., Villani, A. et al (2018) 'Cyberbullying a modern form of bullying: let's talk about this health and social problem', *Italian Journal of Pediatrics*, 44(14). doi: 10.1186/s13052-018-0446-4

Ferry, F., Bolton, D., Bunting, B. et al (2010) 'The experience and psychological impact of "Troubles" related trauma in Northern Ireland', *The Irish Journal of Psychology*, 31(1–4): 95–110.

Ferry, F., Bolton, D., Bunting, B. et al (2011) *The Economic Impact of Post Traumatic Stress Disorder in Northern Ireland*, The Lupina Foundation, Northern Ireland Centre for Trauma & Transformation and University of Ulster.

Fink, D.S., Santaella-Tenorio, J. and Keyes, K.M. (2018) 'Increase in suicides the months after the death of Robin Williams in the US', *PLoS ONE*, 13(2): e0191405.

Fisher, F. (2022) 'Moving social policy from mental illness to public wellbeing', *Journal of Social Policy*, 51(3): 567–81.

Folkman, S. and Lazarus, R.S. (1986) 'Stress processes and depressive symptomatology', *Journal of Abnormal Psychology*, 95(2): 107–13.

Foucault, M. (1961) *Madness and Civilzation: A History of Insanity in the Age of Reason*, Routledge.

Foulkes, L. and Andrews, J.L. (2023) 'Are mental health awareness efforts contributing to the rise in reported mental health problems? A call to test the prevalence inflation hypothesis', *New Ideas in Psychology*, 69: 101010. doi 10.1016/j.newideapsych.2023.101010

Fried, E.I. (2022) 'Studying mental health problems as systems, not syndromes', *Current Directions in Psychological Science*, 31(6): 500–8.

Gabbard, G.O. and Gabbard, K. 'Cinematic stereotypes contributing to the stigmatization of psychiatrists'. In: P.J. Fink and A. Tasman (eds) *Stigma and Mental Illness*, Arlington. VA: American Psychiatric Association. pp. 113–26.

Garcia-Vergara, E., Almeda, N., Martín Ríos, B. et al (2022) 'A comprehensive analysis of factors associated with intimate partner femicide: a systematic review', *International Journal of Environmental Research and Public Health*, 19(12): 7336. doi: 10.3390/ijerph19127336

Garratt, K. (2023) *Mental Health Policy and Services in England*, House of Commons Library Research Briefing [Online], 9 October, Available: https://commonslibrary.parliament.uk/research-briefings/cbp-7547/ (Accessed 13 July 2023).

Garratt, K. and Laing, J. (2022) *Mental Health Policy in England*, House of Commons Library Research Briefing, 6 June, Available: www.mentalhealthlaw.co.uk/Katherine_Garratt_and_Judy_Laing,_%27Reforming_the_Mental_Health_Act%27_(House_of_Commons_Library_research_briefing_CBP-9132,_6/6/22).

Garratt, K., Laing, J. and Long, R. (2022) 'Support for children and young people's mental health (England)', House of Commons Library, 1 June.

Gilburt, H. and Ross, H. (2023) *Actions to Support Partnership: Addressing Barriers to Working with the VCSE Sector in Integrated Care Systems*, London: The King's Fund.

Glasby, J. and Tew, J. (2015) *Interagency Working in Health and Social Care: Mental Health Policy and Practice* (3rd edn), London: Palgrave.

Gnanapragasam, S., Astill Wright, L., Pemberton, M. et al (2023) 'Outside/inside: social determinants of mental health', *Irish Journal of Psychological Medicine*, 40(1): 63–73.

Goffman, E. (1961) *Asylums: Essays on the Social Situation of Mental Patients and Other Inmates*, London: Doubleday.

Goffman, E. (1963) *Stigma: Note on the Management of Spoiled Identity*, Englewood Cliffs, NJ: Prentice-Hall.

Gupta, M. and Sharma, A. (2021) 'Fear of missing out: A brief overview of origin, theoretical underpinnings and relationship with mental health', *World J Clin Cases*, 9(19): 4881–89.

Ha, J. and Yang, H.-S. (2021) 'The Werther effect of celebrity suicides: evidence from South Korea', PLOS ONE, 16(4): e0249896. doi: 10.1371/journal.pone.0249896

Harper, C., Davidson, G. and McClelland, R. (2016) 'No longer "anomalous, confusing and unjust": the Mental Capacity Act (Northern Ireland) 2016', *International Journal of Mental Health and Capacity Law*, 22: 57–70.

Hasan, F., Foster, M.M. and Cho, H. (2023) 'Normalizing anxiety on social media increases self-diagnosis of anxiety: the mediating effect of identification (but not stigma)', *Journal of Health Communication*, 28(9): 563–72.

Hawton, K., Saunders, K.E.A. and O'Connor, R.C. (2012) 'Self-harm and suicide in adolescents', *The Lancet*, 379(9834): 2373–82.

Hayes, D., Camacho, E.M., Ronaldson, A. et al (2023) 'Evidence-based recovery colleges: developing a typology based on organisational characteristics, fidelity and funding', *Social Psychiatry and Psychiatric Epidemiology*, 59: 759–68.

Hayward, P. and Bright, J.A. (1997) 'Stigma and mental illness: a review and critique', *Journal of Mental Health*, 6(4): 345–54.

Hazell, C.M., Berry, C., Bogen-Johnston, L., Banerjee, M. (2022) 'Creating a hierarchy of mental health stigma: testing the effect of psychiatric diagnosis on stigma', *BJPsych Open*. 8(5): e174.

Health Innovation Network (2016) 'What is person-centred care and why is it important' [Online], 22 February, Available: https://healthinnovationnetwork.com/report/what-is-person-centered-care-and-why-is-it-important/?cn-reloaded=1 (Accessed 28 May 2024).

Henderson, C. and Thornicroft, G. (2013) 'Evaluation of the time to change program in England 2008–2011', *The British Journal of Psychiatry*, 202: S45–S48.

Henderson, C. and Gronholm, P.C. (2018) 'Mental health related stigma as a "wicked Problem": the need to address stigma and consider the consequences', *International Journal of Environmental Research and Public Health*, 15(6): 1158. doi: 10.3390/ijerph15061158

Henderson, C., Noblett, J. and Parke, H. (2014) 'Mental health-related stigma in healthcare and mental health–care settings', *The Lancet Psychiatry*, 1(6): 467–82.

Hermaszewska, S., Sweeney, A. and Sin, J. (2022) 'Time to change course in stigma research?', *Journal of Mental Health*, 31(1): 1–4.

Herron, S. and Mortimer, R. (2000) '"Mental health": a contested concept', in M.C. Murray and C.A. Reed (eds) *Promotion of Mental Health* (Vol 7), London: Ashgate.

Hinduja, S. and Patchin, J.W. (2014) *Bullying Beyond the Schoolyard: Preventing and Responding to Cyberbullying* (2nd ed), Thousand Oaks, CA: Corwin.

HL Deb (1962) The Hospital Plan, 14 February, vol 237, cols 472–58.

HM Government (2011) *No Health Without Mental Health: A Cross-Government Mental Health Outcomes Strategy for People of All Ages* [Online], Available: https://assets.publishing.service.gov.uk/gov ernment/uploads/system/uploads/attachment_data/file/213761/ dh_124058.pdf (Accessed 23 April 2023).

HM Government (2017) *Preventing Suicide in England: Third progress report of the cross-government outcomes strategy to save lives* [Online], Available: https://assets.publishing.service.gov.uk/media/5a7ffeaaed915 d74e33f7d24/Suicide_report_2016_A.pdf (Accessed 12 August 2024).

HM Government (2019) *Cross-Government Suicide Prevention Workplan* [Online], Available: https://assets.publishing.service.gov.uk/ media/64fed85157e884000de127e3/DHSC-national-suicide-pre vention-strategy-workplan-accessible-withdrawn.pdf (Accessed 20 July 2024).

HM Government (2021a) *Preventing Suicide in England: Fifth Progress Report of the Cross-Government Outcomes Strategy to Save Lives* [Online], Available: www.gov.uk/government/publications/suicide-prevent ion-in-england-fifth-progress-report (Accessed 20 March 2024).

HM Government (2021b) *Reforming the Mental Health Act* [Online], Available: https://www.gov.uk/government/consultations/reform ing-the-mental-health-act/reforming-the-mental-health-act (Accessed 5 August 2024).

HMSO June 1971 'Better services for the mentally handicapped', Hansard HC Debate. (12 July 1971) Vol 821 cc35.

Hogan, A.J. (2019) 'Social and medical models of disability and mental health: evolution and renewal', *Canadian Medical Association Journal*, 19(1): 16–18.

Holwerda, T.J., Deeg, J.H.D., Beekman, T.F.A. et al (2012) 'Feelings of loneliness, but not social isolation, predict dementia onset: results from the Amsterdam Study of the Elderly (AMSTEL)', *Journal of Neurology, Neurosurgery & Psychiatry*, 85(2): 133–4.

House of Commons Health and Social Care Committee (2021) *The Health and Social Care Committee's Expert Panel: Evaluation of the Government's Progress against its Policy Commitments in the Area of Mental Health Services in England*, [Online], Available: https://publications.parliament.uk/pa/cm5802/cmselect/cmhealth/612/report.html#:~:text=Our%20evaluation%20suggests%20that%20progress,NHS%20Mental%20Health%20Implementation%20Plan (Accessed 20 July 2024).

House of Commons Health Committee (2013) *Pre-Legislative Scrutiny of the Mental Health Act 2007, First Report of Session 2013–2014* [Online], Available: https://publications.parliament.uk/pa/cm201314/cmselect/cmhealth/584/584.pdf (Accessed 20 March 2024).

Huggard, L., Murphy, R., O'Connor, C. et al (2023) 'The social determinants of mental illness: a rapid review of systematic reviews', *Issues in Mental Health Nursing*, 44(4): 302–12.

Human Rights Watch (2019) 'Nigeria: people with mental health conditions chained, abused', *Human Rights Watch* [Online], 11 November, Available: www.hrw.org/news/2019/11/11/nigeria-people-mental-health-conditions-chained-abused#:~:text=In%20some%20cases%2C%20police%20arrest,cases%20for%20months%20or%20years (Accessed 20 July 2024).

Hunt, M.G., Marx, R., Lipson, C. et al (2018) 'No more FOMO: limiting social media decreases loneliness and depression', *Journal of Social and Clinical Psychology*, 37(10): 751–68.

Hussain, Z. and Wegmann, E. (2021) 'Problematic social networking site use and associations with anxiety, attention deficit hyperactivity disorder, and resilience', *Computers in Human Behavior Reports*, doi.org/10.1016/j.chbr.2021.100125

Hyler, S.E., Gabbard, G.O., Schneider, I. (1991) 'Homicidal maniacs and narcissistic parasites: stigmatization of mentally ill persons in the movies', *Hospital and Community Psychiatry*, 42(10): 1044–48.

Institute of Health Metrics and Evaluation (nd) 'Global Health Data Exchange (GHDx)' [Online data], Available: https://vizhub.healthd ata.org/gbd-results/ (Accessed 23 November 2023).

Institute of Medicine (1994) *Reducing Risks for Mental Disorders: Frontiers for Preventive Intervention Research*, Washington, DC: The National Academies Press.

Jenkins, J.H. and Carpenter-Song, E.A. (2008) 'Stigma despite recovery: strategies for living in the aftermath of psychosis', *Medical Anthropology Quarterly*, 22(4): 381–409.

Joint Committee on the Draft Mental Health Bill (2023) *Draft Mental Health Bill 2022, Report of Session 2022–23* [Online], Available: https://publications.parliament.uk/pa/jt5803/jtselect/ jtmentalhealth/696/report.html (Accessed 20 March 2024).

Jones, K. (1993) *Asylums and After: A Revised History of Mental Health Services*, London: Athlone Press.

Jordan, J., McKenna, H., Keeney, S. and Cutcliffe, J. (2011) 'Providing meaningful care: using the experiences of young suicidal men to inform mental health care services, Short Report', Queen's University Belfast, University of Ulster and Public Health Agency.

Karim, F., Oyewande, A.A., Abdalla, L.F. et al 'Social media use and its connection to mental health: a systematic review', *Cureus*, 12(6): e8627. doi: 10.7759/cureus.8627

Kelleher, C.C. (2003) 'Mental health and "the Troubles" in Northern Ireland: implications of civil unrest for health and wellbeing', *Journal of Epidemiology and Community Health*, 57(7): 474–5.

Keyes, K.M., Whitley, R., Fink, D., Santaella and Pirkis, J. (2021) 'The global impact of celebrity suicides: implications for prevention', *World Psychiatry*, 20(1): 144–5.

Kilbourne, A.M., Keyser, D. and Pincus, H.A. (2010) 'Challenges and opportunities in measuring the quality of mental health care', *Canadian Journal of Psychiatry*, 55(9): 549–57.

Killaspy, H. (2006) 'From the asylum to community care: learning from experience', *British Medical Bulletin*, 79–80(1): 245–58.

Kinsella, C. and Kinsella, C. (2015) *Introducing Mental Health: A Practical Guide* (2nd edn), London: Jessica Kingsley Publishers.

Knaak, S., Mantler, E. and Szeto, A. (2017) 'Mental illness-related stigma in healthcare', *Healthcare Management Forum*, 30(2): 111–16.

Knapp, M., McDaid, D. and Parsonage, M. (2011) *Mental Health Promotion and Mental Illness Prevention: The Economic Case* [Online], Available: https://.gov.uk/government/publications/mental-hea lth-promotion-and-mental-illness-prevention-the-economic-case (Accessed 25 March 2024).

Knifton, L. and Inglis, G. (2020) 'Poverty and mental health: policy, practice and research implications', *BJPsych Bulletin*, 44(5): 193–6.

Kondirolli, F. and Sunder, N. (2022) 'Mental health effects of education', *Health Economics*, 31(2): 22–39.

Kovacevic, R. (2021) 'Mental health: lessons learned in 2020 for 2021 and forward', *Investing in Health, World Bank Blogs* [Online], 11 February, Available: https://blogs.worldbank.org/en/health/mental-health-lessons-learned-2020-2021-and-forward (Accessed 20 July 2024).

Kusch, M. (2017) 'Epistemic relativism, scepticism, pluralism', *Synthese*, 194(12): 4687–703.

Laing, R.D. (1960/2010) *Divided Self*, Penguin.

Lannin, D. and Bible, J. (2022) 'Self-stigma of seeking help: a meta-analysis, in D. Vogel and N. Wade (eds) *The Cambridge Handbook of Stigma and Mental Health*, Cambridge: Cambridge University Press, pp 111–142.

Lebowitz, M.S. and Applebaum, P.S. (2019) 'Biomedical explanations of psychopathology and their implications for attitudes and beliefs about mental disorders', *Annual Review of Clinical Psychology*, 15: 555–7.

Lincoln, K.D. (2000) 'Social support, negative social interactions, and psychological well-being', *Social Service Review*, 74: 231–52.

Link, B. and Phelan, J. (2001) 'Conceptualizing stigma', *Annual Review of Sociology*, 27: 363–85.

Liu, X., Liu, T., Zhou, Z. et al (2023) 'The effect of fear of missing out on mental health: differences in different solitude behaviors', *BMC Psychology*, 11: 141. doi: 10.1186/s40359-023-01184-5

Lozito, B. and Horsely, L. (2020) *VCSE Sector and ICS Integration: Evaluation of the NHS England and NHS Improvement's VCSE Leadership Programme*, London: Traverse.

Luca, L., Burlea, S.L., Chirosca, A.C. et al (2020) 'The FOMO syndrome and the perception of personal needs in contemporary society', *BRAIN: Broad Research in Artificial Intelligence and Neuroscience*, 11(suppl 1): 38–46.

Lund, C., Brooke-Sumner, C. and Baingana, F. et al (2018) 'Social determinants of mental disorders and the Sustainable Development Goals: a systematic review of reviews', *The Lancet Psychiatry*, 5(4): 357–69.

Lushey, C., Hyde-Dryden, G., Holmes, L. et al (2017) *Evaluation of the No Wrong Door Innovation Programme*, London: Department for Education.

Lyall, L.M., Wyse, C.A., Graham, N. et al (2018) 'Association of disrupted circadian rhythmicity with mood disorders, subjective wellbeing, and cognitive function: a cross-sectional study of 91 105 participants from the UK Biobank', *The Lancet Psychiatry*, 5(6): 507–51.

Mahomed, F. (2020) 'Addressing the problem of severe underinvestment in mental health and well-being from a human rights perspective', *Health and Human Rights*, 22(1): 35–49.

Mannan, M. and Al-Ghamdi, S.G.I. (2021) 'Indoor air quality in buildings: a comprehensive review on the factors influencing air pollution in residential and commercial structure', *International Journal of Environmental Research and Public Health*, 18(6): 3276. doi: 10.3390/ijerph18063276

Mannarini, S. and Rossi, A. (2019) 'Assessing mental illness stigma: a complex issue', *Frontiers in Psychology*, 9(2722): 1–5.

Marmot, M. (2010) *Fair Society, Healthy Lives: The Marmot Review* [Online], Available: www.instituteofhealthequity.org/resources-repo rts/fair-society-healthy-lives-the-marmot-review/fair-society-heal thy-lives-full-report-pdf.pdf (Accessed 20 July 2024).

Marmot, M. and Bell, R. (2016) 'Social inequalities in health: a proper concern of epidemiology', *Annals of Epidemiology*, 26(4): 238–40.

Masterson, D., Areskoug Josefsson, K., Robert, G. et al (2022) 'Mapping definitions of co-production and co-design in health and social care: a systematic scoping review providing lessons for the future', *Health Expectations*, 25(3): 902–13.

Maurya, C., Muhammad, T. and Dhillon, P. (2022) 'The effects of cyberbullying victimization on depression and suicidal ideation among adolescents and young adults: a three year cohort study from India', *BMC Psychiatry*, 22: 599. doi: 10.1186/s12888-022-04238-x

McDonald, A. (2017) *Invisible Wounds: The Impact of Six Years of War on the Mental Health of Syria's Children*, Save the Children.

Meier, A. and Reinecke, L. (2021) 'Computer-mediated communication, social media, and mental health: a conceptual and empirical meta-review', *Communication Research*, 48(8): 1182–209.

Melzer, D., Fryers, T., Jenkins, R., Brugha, T. and McWilliams, B. (2003) 'Social position and the common mental disorders with disability: estimates from the National Psychiatric Survey of Great Britain', *Social Psychiatry and Psychiatric Epidemiology*, 38(5): 238–43.

Mental Health Foundation (2022) *The Economic Case for Investing in the Prevention of Mental Health Conditions in the UK*, London: Mental Health Foundation.

Mental Health Foundation (2023) *Mental Health and the Cost-of-Living-Crisis: Another Pandemic in the Making?* Glasgow: Mental Health Foundation.

Mental Health Foundation (nd) 'The cost of diagnosed mental health conditions: statistics' [Online], Available: www.mentalhealth.org.uk/explore-mental-health/mental-health-statistics/cost-diagnosed-mental-health-conditions-statistics#:~:text=Mental%20health%20probl ems%20are%20one,the%20overall%20disease%20burden%20worldw ide.&text=Untreated%20mental%20health%20problems%20acco unt,of%20mortality%20and%20morbidity%20globally (Accessed 16 July 2024).

Mental Health Reform (2022) *Resetting the Non-Profit Voluntary & Community (VCS) Mental Health Sector After the Pandemic: A Strategic Perspective*, Dublin: Mental Health Reform.

Mental Health Taskforce (2016) *Five Year Forward View for Mental Health: A Report from the Independent Mental Health Taskforce to the NHS in England* [Online], Available: www.england.nhs.uk/wp-cont ent/uploads/2016/02/Mental-Health-Taskforce-FYFV-final.pdf (Accessed 11 July 2024).

Meshi, D., Elizarova, A., Bender, A. et al (2019) 'Excessive social media users demonstrate impaired decision making in Iowa Gambling Task', *Journal of Behavioral Addictions*, 8(1): 169–73.

Metcalfe, J.D. and Drake, R.E. (2021) 'Participation in Individual Placement and Support in the supported employment demonstration', *Administration and Policy in Mental Health and Mental Health Services Research*, 49: 521–9.

Meyer, M.D., Fallah, A.M. and Wood, M.M. (2011) 'Gender, media, and madness: reading a rhetoric of women in crisis through Foucauldian theory', *Review of Communication*, 11(3), 216–28.

Mikton, C., De la Fuente-Nunez, V., Officer, A. et al (2021) 'Ageism: a social determinant of health that has come of age', *The Lancet*, 397(10282): 1331–4.

Millar, S., Chambers, M. and Giles, M. (2015) 'Service user involvement in mental health care: an evolutionary concept analysis', *Health Expectations*, 19(2): 209–21.

Miller, C., Bubrick, J. and Hamlet, A. (2024) 'Does social media use cause depression?' *Child Mind* [Online]. Available: https://childm ind.org/article/is-social-media-use-causing-depression/

Milner, A., Kavanagh, A., King, T. et al (2018) 'The influence of masculine norms and occupational factors on mental health: evidence from the baseline of the Australian longitudinal study on male health', *American Journal of Men's Health*, 12(4): 696–705.

Mind (2014) 'Mind reveals "unacceptably low" spending on public mental health' [Online], 20 October, Available: www.mind.org.uk/ news-campaigns/news/mind-reveals-unacceptably-low-spending-on-public-mental-health/ (Accessed 15 July 2024).

Mind (2015) 'Mind reveals negligible spend on public mental health' [Online], 9 November, Available: https://www.mind.org.uk/news-campaigns/news/mind-reveals-negligible-spend-on-public-mental-health/ (Accessed 15 July 2024).

Mind (2016) 'The most common diagnosed mental health problems: statistics', [Online]. Available: https://www.mentalhealth.org.uk/explore-mental-health/statistics/most-common-diagnosed-mental-health-problems-statistics (Accessed 22 August 2024).

Mind (nd-a) 'Antidepressants' [Online], Available: www.mind.org.uk/information-support/drugs-and-treatments/antidepressants/about-antidepressants/ (Accessed 9 July 2024).

Mind (nd-b) 'Antipsychotics' [Online], Available: www.mind.org.uk/information-support/drugs-and-treatments/antipsychotics/about-antipsychotics/ (Accessed 9 July 2024).

Mind (2023) 'UK government shelves the Mental Health Bill' [Online], Available: https://www.mind.org.uk/news-campaigns/news/uk-government-shelves-the-mental-health-bill/ (Accessed 6 August 2024).

Moran, P., Coffey, C. and Romaniuk, H. (2012) 'The natural history of self-harm from adolescence to young adulthood: a population-based cohort study', *The Lancet*, 379(9821): 236–43.

Morgan, C., Kirkbride, J., Hutchinson, G. et al (2008) 'Cumulative social disadvantage, ethnicity and first-episode psychosis: a case-control study', *Psychological Medicine*, 38(12): 1701–15.

Morgan, E., Niaz, U., Omigbodun, O. et al (2018) 'The Lancet Commission on global mental health and sustainable development', *The Lancet*, 392(10157): 1553–98.

Mullen, P.E. (2000) 'Forensic mental health', *British Journal of Psychiatry*, 176(4): 307–11.

Mushtaq, R., Shoib, S., Shah, T. et al (2014) 'Relationship between loneliness, psychiatric disorders and physical health? A review on the psychological aspects of loneliness', *Journal of Clinical and Diagnostic Research*, 8(9): WE01–WE04.

Naruse, K. (2023) 'Seven ways social media can benefit mental health', *Painted Brain* [Online], 4 October, Available: https://paintedbrain.org/editorial/7-ways-social-media-can-benefit-mental-health-2 (Accessed 23 November 2023).

Naslund, J.A., Bondre, A., Torous, J. et al (2020) 'Social media and mental health: benefits, risks, and opportunities for research and practice', *Journal of Technology and Behavioral Science*, 5(3): 245–57.

National Alliance on Mental Illness (2012) *Obsessive-Compulsive Disorder Fact Sheet*, Arlington, VA: NAMI.

National Audit Office (2023) *Progress in Improving Mental Health Services in England*, Session 2022–23 [Online], 9 February, Available: www.nao.org.uk/reports/progress-in-improving-mental-health-services-in-england/ (Accessed 15 July 2024).

National Confidential Inquiry into Suicide and Safety in Mental Health (2017) *Annual Report 2017: England, Northern Ireland, Scotland and Wales* [Online], Available: https://sites.manchester.ac.uk/ncish/reports/annual-report-2017-england-northern-ireland-scotland-and-wales/ (Accessed 1 June 2023).

National Confidential Inquiry into Suicide and Safety in Mental Health (2023) *Annual Report 2023: UK Patient and General Population Data 2010-2020* [Online], Available: https://sites.manchester.ac.uk/ncish/reports/annual-report-2023/ (Accessed 2 June 2023).

National Institute of Mental Health (nd) *Bipolar Disorder* [Online], Available: www.nimh.nih.gov/health/publications/bipolar-disorder (Accessed 7 July 2024).

National Records of Scotland (2021) 'Probable suicides 2020' [Online], Available: https://www.nrscotland.gov.uk/files/statistics/probable-suicides/2020/suicides-20-report.pdf (Accessed 6 September 2024).

National Records of Scotland (2022) 'Probable suicides 2021' [Online], Available: https://www.nrscotland.gov.uk/files/statistics/probable-suicides/2021/suicides-21-report.pdf (Accessed 6 September 2024).

National Survivor User Network (2019) 'World Mental Health Day – the crisis of user-led organisations' [Online], 9 October, Available: www.nsun.org.uk/news/world-mental-health-day-the-crisis-of-user-led-organisations/ (Accessed 25 March 2024).

Naylor, C., Parsonage, M., McDaid, D. et al (2012) *Long-Term Conditions and Mental Health: The Cost of Co-Morbidities*, London: The King's Fund and Centre for Mental Health.

Naylor, C., Taggart, H. and Charles, A. (2017) *Mental Health and New Models of Care: Lessons from the Vanguards*, London: The King's Fund and Royal College of Psychiatrists.

NESTA (2013) 'Co-production: right here, right now' [Online], 1 November, Available: www.nesta.org.uk/report/co-production-right-here-right-now/ (Accessed 15 July 2024).

Newbigging, K., Rees, J., Ince, R. et al (2020) 'The contribution of the voluntary sector to mental health crisis care: a mixed-methods study', *Health Services and Delivery Research*, 8(29). doi: 10.3310/hsdr08290

Newman, M.G. and Zainal, N.H. (2020) 'The value of maintaining social connections for mental health in older people', *The Lancet Public Health*, 5(1) e12–e13.

Ngamaba, K.H., Moran, N. and Webber, M. (2023) 'The recovery process and access to social capital of people with severe mental health problems: secondary analysis of a six month follow-up study in England', *Journal of Recovery in Mental Health*, 6(1): 45–64.

NHS (2014) *Five Year Forward View* [Online], Available: www.engl and.nhs.uk/wp-content/uploads/2014/10/5yfv-web.pdf (Accessed 10 June 2023).

NHS (2019) *The NHS Long Term Plan* [Online], Available: www.longtermplan.nhs.uk/wp-content/uploads/2019/08/nhs-long-term-plan-version-1.2.pdf (Accessed 15 July 2024).

NHS Digital (2022a) *Mental Health Bulletin, 2021–22 Annual Report* [Online], Available: https://digital.nhs.uk/data-and-info rmation/publications/statistical/mental-health-bulletin (Accessed 14 March 2024).

NHS Digital (2022b) 'Mental Health of Children and Young People in England 2022 – wave 3 follow up to the 2017 survey', [Online], 29 November, Available: https://digital.nhs.uk/data-and-informat ion/publications/statistical/mental-health-of-children-and-young-people-in-england (Accessed 25 March 2024).

NHS Digital (2023) 'A&E relating to self-harm', 3 February 2023 [Online]. Available: https://digital.nhs.uk/supplementary-information/2023/ae-attendances-relating-to-self-harm

NHS Digital (nd-a) 'Learning disability services statistics' [Online], Available: https://digital.nhs.uk/data-and-information/publi cations/statistical/learning-disability-services-statistics (Accessed 13 July 2024).

NHS Digital (nd-b) 'Psychological therapies, annual reports on the use of IAPT services' [Online], Available: https://digital.nhs.uk/data-and-information/publications/statistical/psychological-therapies-annual-reports-on-the-use-of-iapt-services (Accessed 14 March 2023).

NHS England (2019a) *NHS Mental Health Implementation Plan 2019/20-2023/24* [Online], Available: www.longtermplan.nhs.uk/publication/nhs-mental-health-implementation-plan-2019-20-2023-24/ (Accessed 19 July 2024).

NHS England (2019b) *The Community Mental Health Framework for Adults and Older Adults* [Online], Available: www.england.nhs.uk/publication/the-community-mental-health-framework-for-adults-and-older-adults/ (Accessed 10 June 2023).

NHS England (2022) *Care Programme Approach: NHS Position Statement*, Version 2.0 [Online], 1 March, Available: www.england.nhs.uk/publication/care-programme-approach-position-statement/#:~:text=It%20enables%20services%20to%20shift,need%20of%20community%20mental%20healthcare (Accessed 25 March 2024).

NHS England (2023) *A Framework for addressing practical barriers to integration of VCSE organisations in integrated care systems* [Online]. Available: https://www.england.nhs.uk/long-read/a-framework-for-addressing-practical-barriers-to-integration-of-vcse-organisations-in-integrated-care-systems/ (Accessed 6 September 2024).

NHS England (nd-a) 'NHS Talking Therapies, for anxiety and depression' [Online], Available: www.england.nhs.uk/mental-health/adults/nhs-talking-therapies/ (Accessed 14 March 2023).

NHS England (nd-b) 'Person-centred care' [Online], Available: www.hee.nhs.uk/our-work/person-centred-care#:~:text=carers%20are%20identified%2C%20supported%20and,are%20recognised%20as%20key%20enablers (Accessed 19 July 2024).

NHS England and NHS Health Improvement (2021) *Building Strong Integrated Care Systems Everywhere: ICS Implementation Guidance on Partnerships with the Voluntary, Community and Social Enterprise Sector*, Version 1 [Online], 2 September, Available: www.england.nhs.uk/wp-content/uploads/2021/06/B0905-vcse-and-ics-partnerships.pdf (Accessed 25 March 2024).

NHS Health Education England (2017) 'Person-centred approaches: Empowering people in their lives and communities to enable an upgrade in prevention, wellbeing, health, care and support', [Online] Available: www.skillsforhealth.org.uk/wp-content/uploads/2021/01/Person-Centred-Approaches-Framework.pdf (Accessed 12 August 2024).

NHS Surrey and Borders Partnership NHS Foundation Trust (nd-a) 'A new vision for community mental health services' [Online] Available: www.sabp.nhs.uk/aboutus/services-and-site-developments/transformation-community-mental-health-services (Accessed 30 April 2023).

NHS Surrey and Borders Partnership NHS Foundation Trust (nd-b) 'The transformation of community mental health services' [Online], Available: www.sabp.nhs.uk/aboutus/our-trust/services-and-site-developments/transformation-community-mental-health-services (Accessed 27 February 2024).

NICCY (Northern Ireland Commissioner for Children and Young People) (2018) *Still Waiting: A Rights Based Review of Mental Health Services and Support for Children and Young People in Northern Ireland*, Belfast: NICCY.

NICE (National Institute for Health and Care Excellence) (2016) 'Transition between inpatient mental health settings and community care or care home settings' [Online], Available: www.nice.org.uk/guidance/ng53/resources/tailored-resources-4429245855/chapter/3-co-producing-comprehensive-care-plans-that-meet-peoples-changing-needs (Accessed 19 July 2024).

Niederkrotenthaler, T., Voracek, M. and Herberth, A. (2010) 'Role of media reports in completed and prevented suicide: Werther v. Papageno effects', *British Journal of Psychiatry*, 197: 234–43.

Northern Ireland Audit Office (2023) *Mental Health Services in Northern Ireland*, Belfast: NIAO.

Northern Ireland Statistical Research Agency (NISRA) (2022) 'Suicide statistics 2021' [Online], Available: https://www.nisra.gov.uk/publications/suicide-statistics-2021 (Accessed 6 September 2024).

Nuffield Trust (2021) 'Suicide in mental health service users' [Online], Available: www.nuffieldtrust.org.uk/resource/suicide-in-mental-health-service-users (Accessed 20 July 20024).

Nuffield Trust (2022) 'NHS Talking Therapies (IAPT) programme' [Online], last updated 4 May 2022, Available: www.nuffieldtrust.org.uk/resource/improving-access-to-psychological-therapies-iapt-programme (Accessed 23 February 2023).

OECD (Organisation for Economic Co-operation and Development) (2021) *Fitter Minds, Fitter Jobs: From Awareness to Change in Integrated Mental Health, Skills and Work Policies*, Paris: OECD Publishing.

Office for National Statistics (nd) 'Stalking: findings from the Crime Survey for England and Wales' [Online dataset], Available: www.ons.gov.uk/peoplepopulationandcommunity/crimeandjustice/datasets/stalkingfindingsfromthecrimesurveyforenglandandwales (Accessed 23 July 2024).

Office for National Statistics (2022) 'Suicides in England and Wales: 2021 Registrations', [Online] Available: www.ons.gov.uk/peoplepopulationandcommunity/birthsdeathsandmarriages/deaths/bulletins/suicidesintheunitedkingdom/2021registrations

O'Neill, S., Heenan, D. and Betts, J. (2019) *Review of Mental Health Policies in Northern Ireland: Making Parity a Reality* [Online], Available: www.ulster.ac.uk/__data/assets/pdf_file/0004/452155/Final-Draft-Mental-Health-Review-web.pdf (Accessed 9 June 2023).

O'Reilly, M., Dogra, N., Whiteman, N. et al (2018) 'Is social media bad for mental health and wellbeing? Exploring the perspectives of adolescents', *Clinical Child Psychology Psychiatry*, 23(4): 601–13.

O'Sullivan, M. and Tiernan, E. (eds) (2023) *Suicide Prevention in the Community: Connecting, Communicating Caring. A Practical Guide*, Dublin: HSE National Office for Suicide Prevention.

Owen, P.R. (2012) 'Portrayals of schizophrenia by entertainment media: a content analysis of contemporary movies', *Psychiatric Services*, 63(7): 655–9.

Oxford English Dictionary (2022) 'Stigma'.

Palermiti, A., Servidio, R. and Bartolo, M.G. (2017) 'Cyberbullying and self-esteem: an Italian study', *Computer Human Behaviour*, 69: 136–41.

Papadimitriou, G. (2017) 'The "biopsychosocial model": 40 years of application in Psychiatry', *Psychiatriki*, 28: 107–10.

Parker, H.W., Abreu, A.M., Sullivan, M.C. et al (2022) 'Allostatic load and mortality: a systematic review and meta-analysis', *American Journal of Preventive Medicine*, 63(1): 131–40.

Parker, M., Bucknall, M., Jaggar, C. et al (2020) 'Population-based estimates of healthy working life expectancy in England at age 50 years: analysis of data from English Longitudinal Study of Ageing', *The Lancet Public Health*, 5(7): 395–403.

Patel, V., Saxena, S., Lund, C. et al (2018) 'The Lancet Commission on global mental health and sustainable development', *The Lancet*, 392(10157): 1553–98. [Erratum in: *The Lancet*, 2018, 392(10157): 1518.]

Patel, V., Saxena, S., Lund, C. et al (2023) 'Transforming mental health systems globally: principles and policy recommendations', *The Lancet*, 402(10402): 656–66.

Patton, G.C., Darmstadt, G.L., Petroni, S. et al (2018) 'A gender lens on the health and well-being of young males', *Journal of Adolescent Health*, 62: S6–S8.

Pavelko, R.L. and Myrick, J.G. (2015) 'That's so OCD: the effects of disease trivialisation via social media on user perceptions and impression formation', *Computers in Human Behaviour*, 49: 251–8.

Pavelko, R. and Myrick, J.G. (2016) 'Tweeting and trivializing: how the trivialization of obsessive-compulsive disorder via social media impacts user perceptions, emotions, and behaviours', *Imagination, Cognition and Personality*, 36(1): 41–63.

Perkins, R., Repper, J., Rinaldi, M. et al (2012) *Recovery Colleges*, London: Centre for Mental Health.

Perkins, R., Meddings, S., Williams, S. et al (2018) *Recovery Colleges 10 Years On*, Nottingham: ImROC.

Perloff, R.M. (2014) 'Social media effects on young women's body image concerns: theoretical perspectives and an agenda for research', *Sex Roles*, 71(11–12): 363–77.

Phillips, D.P. (1974) 'The influence of suggestion on suicide: substantive and theoretical implications of the Werther effect', *American Sociological Review*, 39: 340–54.

Pieper, K., Khan, A.B., Case, A. et al (2023) *Mental Health Conditions Across 300 Popular Films: A Research Update from 2016–2022* [Online], Available: https://assets.uscannenberg.org/docs/aii-mental-health-2023-06-28.pdf (Accessed 20 July 2024).

Pilgrim, D. (2017) *Key Concepts in Mental Health* (4th edn), Sage: London.

Pilgrim, D. (2002) 'The biopsychosocial model in Anglo-American psychiatry, past, present and future', *Journal of Mental Health*, 11(6): 585–94.

Pilgrim, D. and Waldron, L. (1998) 'User involvement in mental health services: how far can it go?', *Journal of Mental Health*, 7(1): 95–104.

Porter, R. (1985) 'The patient's view: doing medical history from below', *Theory and Society*, 14(2): 175–98.

Porter, R. (2002) *Madness: A Brief History*, Oxford: Oxford University Press.

Powell, E. (1961) 'Official opening of the conference', National Association for Mental Health conference, London, 9–10 March, in *The Speeches of Enoch Powell*, POLL 4/1/1 [Online], Available: http://enochpowell.info/wp-content/uploads/Speeches/1957-1961.pdf (Accessed 11 July 2024).

Powers, R.A. (2015) *Poor Education: The Social Determinants of Mental Health*, Arlington, VA: American Psychiatric Publishing.

Prince's Trust (2018) *Youth Index 2018*, Prince's Trust and MacQuarie Group.

Prior, P. (1993) 'Mental health policy in Northern Ireland', *Social Policy & Administration*, 27(4): 323–34.

Prnjak, K., Hay, P., Mond, J., Bussey, K., Trompeter, N., Lonergan, A. and Mitchison, D. (2021) 'The distinct role of body image aspects in predicting eating disorder onset in adolescents after one year', *Journal of Abnormal Psychology*, 130(3): 236–47.

The Public Health Agency (2022) 'Northern Ireland Registry of Self-Harm Summary Regional Report, 2019/20' [Online], Available: https://niopa.qub.ac.uk/bitstream/NIOPA/16586/5/NIRSH_Regional_Summary_Report_2019.20.pdf (Accessed 6 September 2024).

Public Health Wales (2018) 'Midpoint review of the implementation of Talk to me 2: the Wales suicide and self-harm prevention action plan' [Online], Available: https://www.gov.wales/sites/default/files/publications/2020-08/suicide-and-self-harm-prevention-strategy-2015-to-2020-mid-point-review.pdf (Accessed 12 August 2024).

Queensland Brain Institute (2023) 'Half of the world's population will experience a mental health disorder'. Available: https://hms.harvard.edu/news/half-worlds-population-will-experience-mental-health-disorder (Accessed 21 August 2024).

Race Equality Foundation (2022) *Collaboratives on Addressing Racial Inequity in Covid Recovery*, Mental Health Briefing Paper [Online], Available: https://raceequalityfoundation.org.uk/wp-content/uploads/2022/12/collaborative-briefing-mental-health-briefing-digital-FINAL.pdf (Accessed 20 July 2024).

Recovery in the Bin (nd) 'About' [Online], Available: https://recoveryinthebin.org/ (Accessed 25 May 2023).

Reer, F., Tang, W.Y. and Quandt, T. (2019) 'Psychosocial well-being and social media engagement: the mediating roles of social comparison orientation and fear of missing out', *New Media & Society*, 21(7): 1486–505.

Research Into Recovery (nd) *RECOLLECT Fidelity Measure for Recovery Colleges* [Online], Available: www.researchintorecovery.com/files/RECOLLECT%20Fidelity%20Measure.pdf (Accessed 25 May 2023).

Rethink Mental Illness (2021) 'Overwhelming majority of people severely affected by mental illness report discrimination still widespread', [Online], 6 May, Available: www.rethink.org/news-and-stories/media-centre/2021/05/new-survey-reveals-overwhelming-majority-88-of-people-severely-affected-by-mental-illness-report-discrimination-still-widespread/#:~:text=New%20survey%20reveals%20overwhelming%20majority,the%20charity%20Rethink%20Mental%20Illness (Accessed 20 July 2024).

Reuben, A. and Schaefer, J. (2017) 'Mental illness is far more common than we knew', *Scientific American*, 14 July [Blog], Available: www.sci entificamerican.com/blog/observations/mental-illness-is-far-more-common-than-we-knew/ (Accessed 15 July 2024).

Rice, S., Oliffe, J., Seidler, Z. et al (2021) 'Gender norms and the mental health of boys and young men', *The Lancet Public Health*, 6(8): 541–42.

Richter, D. and Dixon, J. (2023) 'Models of mental health problems: a quasi-systematic review of theoretical approaches', *Journal of Mental Health*, 32(2): 396–406.

Roberts, G. and Boardman, J. (2013) 'Understanding "recovery"', *Advances in Psychiatric Treatment*, 19(6): 400–9.

Robinson, P., Turk, D., Sagar, J. et al (2019) 'Measuring attitudes towards mental health using social media: investigating stigma and trivialisation', *Social Psychiatry and Psychiatric Epidemiology*, 54: 51–8.

Rogers, A. and Pilgrim, D. (2003) *Mental Health and Inequality*, London: Macmillan Education.

Rosa, G.S.D., Andrades, G.S., Caye, A. et al (2019) 'Thirteen reasons why: the impact of suicide portrayal on adolescents' mental health', *Journal of Psychiatric Research*, 108: 2–6.

Rössler, W. (2016) 'The stigma of mental disorders', *EMBO Reports*, 17(9): 1250–3.

Royal College of Paediatrics and Child Health (2018) 'RCPCH Ireland responds to NICCY' "Still Waiting" review' [Online] Available at: https://www.rcpch.ac.uk/news-events/news/rcpch-irel and-responds-niccys-still-waiting-review (Accessed 6 August 2024).

Royal College of Paediatrics and Child Health (2020) *State of Child Health in the UK* [Online], Available: https://stateofchildhealth. rcpch.ac.uk (Accessed 26 March 2024).

Royal College of Paediatrics and Child Health (nd) 'Prevalence of mental health conditions' [Online], Available: https://stateofchildhealth.rcpch. ac.uk/evidence/mental-health/prevalence/ (Accessed 16 July 2024).

Royal College of Psychiatrists (RCPsych) (2020) *CR229. Self-harm and suicide in adults: Final report of the Patient Safety Group July 2020* [Online], Available: https://www.rcpsych.ac.uk/improving-care/ campaigning-for-better-mental-health-policy/college-reports/2020-college-reports/cr229 (Accessed 6 September 2024).

Royal College of Psychiatrists (nd) *No Wrong Door: The RCPsych in Scotland's Priorities for the 2021–26 Scottish Parliament* [Online], Available: www.rcpsych.ac.uk/docs/default-source/members/divisions/scotland/rcpsychis---manifesto2021---251120.pdf (Accessed 19 April 2023).

Rüsch, N., Angermeyer, M.C., and Corrigan, P.W. (2005) 'Mental illness stigma: concepts, consequences, and initiatives to reduce stigma', *European Psychiatry*, 20(8): 529–39.

Samaritans (nd) 'Samaritans' media guidelines' [Online], Available: www.samaritans.org/about-samaritans/media-guidelines/ (Accessed 26 March 2024).

Saphire-Bernstein, S. and Taylor, S.E. (2013) 'Close relationships and happiness', in S.A. David, I. Boniwell and A. Conley Ayers (eds) *The Oxford Handbook of Happiness*, Oxford: Oxford University Press, pp 821–33.

Saraceno, B. and Barbui, C. (1997) 'Poverty and mental illness', *The Canadian Journal of Psychiatry*, 42(3): 285–90.

Scarf, D., Zimmerman, H., Winter, T. et al (2020) 'Association of viewing the films Joker or Terminator: Dark Fate with prejudice toward individuals with mental illness', *JAMA Network Open*, 3(4): e2034323. doi: 10.1001/jamanetworkopen.2020.3423

Schofield, P., Das-Munshi, J., Webb, R.T. et al (2023) 'Lack of fit with the neighbourhood social environment as a risk factor for psychosis – a national cohort study', *Psychological Medicine*, 53(3): 866–74.

SCIE (Social Care Institute for Excellence) (2020) *Oxfordshire County Council Co-Production in Adult Social Care: Evaluation Report*, London: SCIE.

Science Museum (2019) '"Heroic therapies" in psychiatry' [Online], 13 June, Available: www.sciencemuseum.org.uk/objects-and-stories/medicine/heroic-therapies-psychiatry (Accessed 9 February 2023).

Scottish Government (2002) Choose Life: A National Strategy and Action Plan to Prevent Suicide in Scotland.

Scottish Government (2013) Suicide Prevention Strategy 2013–2016.

Scottish Government (2018) *Every Life Matters: Scotland's Suicide Prevention Action Plan* [Online], Available: www.gov.scot/publicati ons/scotlands-suicide-prevention-action-plan-life-matters/docume nts/ (Accessed 20 March 2024).

Scottish Government (2022a) *The Scottish Health Survey 2021: Volume 1,* [Online], Available: https://www.gov.scot/publications/ scottish-health-survey-2021-volume-1-main-report/ (Accessed 24 November 2024).

Scottish Government (2022b) *Making Suicide Prevention Everyone's Business: Because Together We Can Save Lives. The Fourth Annual Report of the National Suicide Prevention Group* [Online], Available: www.gov. scot/publications/national-suicide-prevention-leadership-group-nsplg-fourth-annual-report/ (Accessed 7 April 2023).

Scottish Government (2022c) *Creating Hope Together: Scotland's Suicide Prevention Strategy 2022–2032* [Online], Available: www.gov.scot/ publications/creating-hope-together-scotlands-suicide-prevention-strategy-2022-2032/ (Accessed 7 April 2023).

Scottish Mental Health Law Review (2022) Final Report [Online] Available at: https://webarchive.nrscotland.gov.uk/20230327160 310/https://cms.mentalhealthlawreview.scot/wp-content/uploads/ 2022/09/SMHLR-FINAL-Report-.pdf (Accessed 9 August 2024).

Scull, A. (2021) 'UK deinstitutionalisation: neoliberal values and mental health', in G. Ikkos and N. Bouras (eds) *Mind, State and Society: Social History of Psychiatry in Britain 1960–2010,* Cambridge: Cambridge University Press, pp 306–14.

Sharek, D., Lally, N., Brennan, C. et al (2022) 'These are people just like us who can work: overcoming clinical resistance and shifting views in the implementation of Individual Placement and Support (IPS)', *Administration and Policy in Mental Health,* 49: 848–60.

Shim, R.S. and Compton, M.T. (2020) 'The social determinants of mental health: psychiatrists' roles in addressing discrimination and food insecurity', *FOCUS. The Journal of Lifelong Learning in Psychiatry,* 18(1): 25–30.

Shipman, C. (1995) *Mental Health Promotion: A Review of Evaluations and Activities,* North Buckinghamshire Health Promotion Unit.

Sintonen, S. and Pehkonen, A. (2014) 'Effect of social networks and well-being on acute care needs', *Health and Social Care in the Community*, 22(1): 87–95.

Skryabin, V. (2021) 'Analysing *Joker*: an attempt to establish diagnosis for a film icon', *BJPsych Bulletin*, 45(6): 329–32.

Slade, M., Bird, V., Le Boutillier, C. et al (2018) *Development of the REFOCUS Intervention to Increase Mental Health Team Support for Personal Recovery*, Cambridge: Cambridge University Press.

South Carolina Department of Mental Health (nd) 'Eating disorder statistics' [Online], Available: www.state.sc.us/dmh/anorexia/statist ics.htm (Accessed 6 February 2023).

Srivastava, K., Chaudhury, S., Bhat, P.S. et al (2018) 'Media and mental health', *Industrial Psychiatry Journal*, 27(1): 1–5.

Statistica (2024) Mental health in the United Kingdom (UK) statistics and facts. https://www.statista.com/topics/8164/mental-health-in-the-uk/#:~:text=One%20in%20four%20adults%20suffers,from%20 seeking%20care%20and%20treatment (Accessed 9 January 2024).

Stuart, H. (2016) 'Reducing the stigma of mental illness', *Global Mental Health*, 3: 1–14.

Subu, M.A., Wati, D.F. and Netrida, N. (2021) 'Types of stigma experienced by patients with mental illness and mental health nurses in Indonesia: a qualitative content analysis', *International Journal of Mental Health Systems*, 15: 77. doi: 10.1186/s13033-021-00502-x

Suler, J. (2004) 'The online disinhibition effect', *Cyberpsychology and Behaviour*, 7(3): 321–6.

Summergrad, P. (2016) 'Investing in global mental: the time for action is now', *The Lancet Psychiatry*, 3(5): 390–1.

Sweeney, A. and Taggart, D. (2018) '(Mis)understanding trauma-informed approaches in mental health', *Journal of Mental Health*, 27(5): 383–7.

Szasz, T. (1961) *The Myth of Mental Illness: Foundations of a Theory of Personal Conduct*, New York: Harper and Row.

Tang, S., Reilly, N., Arena, A. et al (2021) 'People who die by suicide without receiving mental health services: a systematic review', *Frontiers Public Health*, 9: 736948. doi: 10.3389/fpubh.2021.736948

Tew, J. (2015) 'Towards a socially situated model of mental distress', in H. Spandler, J. Anderson and B. Sapey (eds) *Madness, Distress and the Politics of Disablement*, Bristol: Policy Press, pp 69–82.

Thai, H., Davis, C.G., Mahboob, W. et al (2023) 'Reducing social media use improves appearance and weight esteem in youth with emotional distress', *Psychology of Popular Media*, 13(1), 162–9.

The King's Fund (2013) *Co-Ordinated Care for People with Complex Chronic Conditions: Key Lessons and Markers for Success* [Online], Available: www.kingsfund.org.uk/publications/co-ordinated-care-people-complex-chronic-conditions (Accessed 10 June 2023).

The King's Fund (2019) 'Mental health: our position' [Online], Available: https://kingsfund.org.uk/projects/positions/mental-health (Accessed 6 November 2023).

The Lancet Global Health (2020) 'Mental health hatters' [editorial], *The Lancet Global Health*, 8(11): e1352. doi: 10.1016/S2214-109X(20)30432-0

Thibodeau, R. (2020) 'Continuum belief, categorical belief, and depression stigma: correlational evidence and outcomes of an online intervention', *Stigma and Health*, 5(4): 404–12.

Thornicroft, G. (2006) *Shunned: Discrimination against People with Mental Illness*, Oxford: Oxford University Press.

Thornicroft, G. (2011) 'Physical health disparities and mental illness: the scandal of premature mortality', *British Journal of Psychiatry*, 199(6): 441–2.

Thornicroft, G., Mehta, N., Clement, S., Evans-Lacko, S., Doherty, M., Rose, D., Koschorke, M., Shidhaye, R., O'Reilly, C. and Henderson, C. (2016) 'Evidence for effective interventions to reduce mental-health-related stigma and discrimination', *Lancet*. 387(10023): 1123–32.

Tracey, D.K., Holloway, F., Hanson, K. et al (2023) 'Why care about integrated care? Part 1. Demographics, finances and workforce: immovable objects facing mental health services', *BJPsych Advances*, 29: 8–18.

Tse, J.S.Y. and Haslam, N. (2023) 'Individual differences in the expansiveness of mental disorder concepts: development and validation of concept breadth scales', *BMC Psychiatry*, 23: 718. doi: 10.1186/s12888-023-05152-6

Tucker, L., Webber, M. and Jobling, H. (2022) 'Mapping the matrix: understanding the structure and position of social work in mental health services in England and Wales', *British Journal of Social Work*, 52(6): 3210–29.

Turner, J., Hayward, R., Angel, K. et al (2015) 'The history of mental health services in modern England: practitioner memories and the direction of future research', *Medical History*, 59(4): 599–624.

Ulster University (2015) *Towards a Better Future: The Trans-Generational Impact of the Troubles on Mental Health?*, Belfast: Commission for Victims and Survivors.

United Nations (2019) *Global Humanitarian Overview 2019*, Geneva: United Nations.

Vahedi, Z. and Zannella, L. (2021) 'The association between self-reported depressive symptoms and the use of social networking sites: a meta-analysis', *Current Psychology*, 40: 2174–89.

Valkenburg, P.M. (2022) 'Social media use and well-being: what we know and what we need to know', *Current Opinion in Psychology*, 45: 101294. doi: 10.1016/j.copsyc.2021.12.006

Van Geel, M., Vedder, P. and Tanilon, J. (2014) 'Relationship between peer victimization, cyberbullying, and suicide in children and adolescents a meta-analysis', *JAMA Pediatrics*, 168(5): 435–42.

Vigo, D., Jones, L., Atun, R. et al (2022) 'The true global disease burden of mental illness: still elusive', *The Lancet Psychiatry*, 9(2): 98–100.

Vojak, C. (2009) 'Choosing language: social service framing and social justice', *British Journal of Social Work*, 39(5): 936–49.

Wallcraft, J. and Bryant, M. (2003) *The Mental Health Service User Movement in England*, Policy Paper 2, London: Sainsbury Centre for Mental Health.

Wallcraft, J. and Hopper, K. (2015) 'The capabilities model and the social model of mental health', in H. Spandler, J. Anderson and B. Sapey (eds) *Madness, Distress and the Politics of Disablement*, Bristol: Policy Press, pp 83–8.

Walsh, D. and Foster, J. (2021) 'A call to action: a critical review of mental health related anti-stigma campaigns', *Frontiers in Public Health*, 8: 569539. doi: 10.3389/fpubh.2020.569539

Warr, P. (1987) *Work, Unemployment, and Mental Health*, Oxford: Oxford University Press.

Watkins, L.E., Sprang, K.R. and Rothbaum, B.O. (2018) 'Treating PTSD: a review of evidence-based psychotherapy interventions', *Frontiers in Behavioural Neuroscience*, 12: 258. doi: 10.3389/fnbeh.2018.00258

Weiner, B. (1995) *Judgments of Responsibility: A Foundation for a Theory of Social Conduct*, New York: The Guilford Press.

Welsh Government (2009) *Talk to me*, Cardiff: Welsh Government.

Welsh Government (2015) *Talk to me 2: Suicide and Self-Harm Prevention Strategy for Wales 2015-2020* [Online] Available: https://www.gov.wales/sites/default/files/publications/2019-06/talk-to-me-2-suicide-and-self-harm-prevention-action-plan-for-wales-2015-2020.pdf (Accessed 12 August 2024).

Whitley, R., Palmer, V. and Gunn, J. (2015) 'Recovery from severe mental illness', *Canadian Medical Association Journal*, 187(13): 951–2.

WHO (World Health Organization) (2000) *Mental and Behavioral Disorders*, Geneva: WHO.

WHO (World Health Organization) (2008) *Closing the Gap in a Generation*, Final Report of the Commission on Social Determinants for Health, Geneva: WHO.

WHO (World Health Organization) (2001) *The World Health Report: 2001*, Geneva: WHO.

WHO (World Health Organization) (2012) *WHO QualityRights Toolkit: Assessing and Improving Quality and Human Rights in Mental Health and Social Care Facilities* [Online], Available: www.who.int/publications/i/item/9789241548410#:~:text=The%20WHO%20QualityRights%20tool%20kit,Rights%20of%20Persons%20with%20Disabilities (Accessed 21 March 2024).

WHO (World Health Organization) (2014a) *Mental Health: A State of Wellbeing*, Geneva: WHO.

WHO (World Health Organization) (2014b) *Mental Health Atlas 2014*, Geneva: WHO.

WHO (World Health Organization) (2014c) *Review of the Social Determinants and the Health Divide in the WHO European Region* [Online, updated reprint], Available: https://iris.who.int/bitstream/handle/10665/108636/9789289000307-eng.pdf?sequence=1 (Accessed 22 July 2024).

WHO (World Health Organization) (2021a) *Global Report on Ageism* [Online], Available: www.who.int/teams/social-determinants-of-health/demographic-change-and-healthy-ageing/combatting-ageism/global-report-on-ageism (Accessed 20 July 2024).

WHO (World Health Organization) (2021b) *Guidance on Community Mental Health Services: Promoting Person-Centred and Rights-Based Approaches*, Geneva: WHO.

WHO (World Health Organization) (2022a) 'Mental disorders' [Online], 8 June, Available: www.who.int/news-room/fact-sheets/detail/mental-disorders (Accessed 12 March 2024).

WHO (World Health Organization) (2022b) 'Mental health' [Online], 17 June, Available: www.who.int/news-room/fact-sheets/detail/mental-health-strengthening-our-response (Accessed 12 March 2024).

WHO (World Health Organization) (2022c) *World Mental Health Report: Transforming Mental Health for All*, Geneva: WHO.

WHO (World Health Organization) (2023) 'Suicide' [Online]. Available: https://www.who.int/news-room/fact-sheets/detail/suicide (Accessed 6 September 2024).

WHO (World Health Organization) (2024) *Operational Framework for Monitoring Social Determinants of Health Equity*, Geneva: WHO.

WHO (World Health Organization) (nd) 'Health and well-being' [Online], Available: www.who.int/data/gho/data/major-themes/health-and-well-being (Accessed 20 July 2024).

WHO (World Health Organization) and International Association for Suicide Prevention (2017) *Preventing Suicide: A Resource for Media Professionals. Update 2017* [Online], Available: https://iris.who.int/bitstream/handle/10665/258814/WHO-MSD-MER-17.5-eng.pdf?sequence=1#:~:text=Photographs%2C%20video%20footage%20or%20social%20media%20links%20of%20the%20scene,of%20the%20location%20or%20method (Acessed 20 July 2024).

WHO (World Health Organization) Department of Reproductive Health and Research, London School of Hygiene and Tropical Medicine, South African Medical Research Council (2013) 'Global and regional estimates of violence against women: prevalence and health impacts of intimate partner violence and non-partner sexual violence', Geneva, WHO.

Williams, A. (2019) 'We need to stop making mental illness look cool on social media', *Vice* [Online], 17 August. Available: www.vice.com/en/article/a35de4/we-need-to-stop-making-mental-illness-look-cool-on-social-media (Accessed on 20 July 2024).

Williams, A.R. and Caplan, A.L. (2012) 'Thomas Szasz: rebel with a questionable cause', *The Lancet*, 380 (9851): 1378–9.

Williams, D.R., Neighbors, H.W. and Jackson, J.S. (2003) 'Racial/ethnic discrimination and health: findings from community studies', *American Journal of Public Health*, 93(2): 200–8.

Williams, N. (2023) 'How does education affect Mental Health?', *News Medical and Life Sciences* [Online], Available: https://news-medical.net/health/How-does-Education-Affect-Mental-Health.aspx (Accessed 28 May 2024).

Wing, J.K. and Brown, G.W. (1970) *Institutionalism and Schizophrenia*, London and New York: Cambridge University Press.

Wolke, D., Lee, K. and Guy, A. (2017) 'Cyberbullying: a storm in a teacup?', *European Child & Adolescent Psychiatry*, 26: 899–908.

Wood, L., Birtel, M., Alsawy, S. et al (2014) 'Public perceptions of stigma towards people with schizophrenia, depression, and anxiety', *Psychiatry Research*, 220(1–2): 604–8.

World Bank (2016) 'Psychosocial support in fragile and conflict affected settings' [Online], 9 May, Available: https://worldbank.org/en/topic/fragilityconflictviolence/brief/psychosocial-support-in-fragile-and-conflict-affected-settings (Accessed 28 May 2024).

World Economic Forum (2023) *The Global Risks Report 2023: 18th Edition*, Geneva: World Economic Forum.

Wren-Lewis, S. and Alexandrova, A. (2021) 'Mental health without well-being', *Journal of Medicine and Philosophy*, 46(6): 684–703.

Wu, Y.-T., Daskalopoulou, C., Sanchez Niubo, A. et al (2020) 'Education and wealth inequalities in healthy ageing: a population-based study of eight harmonised cohorts in the Ageing Trajectories of Health: Longitudinal Opportunities and Synergies' (ATHLOS) consortium', *The Lancet Public Health*, 5(7): 386–94.

Yan, Y. and Williams, D.R. (1999) 'Socioeconomic status and mental health', in C.S. Aneshensel and J.C. Phelan (eds) *Handbook of the Sociology of Mental Health*, New York: Kluwer Academic/Plenum Publishers, pp 151–66.

Zsila, Á. and Reyes, M.E.S. (2023) 'Pros & cons: impacts of social media on mental health', *BMC Psychology*, 11(1): 201. doi: 10.1186/s40359-023-01243-x

Zubair, U., Khan, M.K. and Albashari, M. (2023) 'Link between excessive social media use and psychiatric disorders', *Annals of Medicine and Surgery*, 85(4): 875–8.

Index